After the Diagnosis...

After the Diagnosis...

A Guide for Living

The Transformative Power of Love
During Sickness, Dying, and Death

Reverend Thomas F. Lynch and Barbara Mariconda

Contact the authors for conferences, workshops,
presentations, programs,
and additional resource materials at
www.journeyofthesoulbooks.com

Copyright ©2018 Reverend Thomas F. Lynch and Barbara Mariconda
Create Space
ISBN-13: 9781981230457
ISBN-10: 1981230459

Praise for *After the Diagnosis: A Guide for Living*

...Lynch and Mariconda's broad-based, narrative-driven work ranges from absorbing accounts of encounters with dying men and women...to engaging meditations on the human reluctance to think about death. The string of personal anecdotes well-illustrates the variety of reactions people have when encountering the final months of their lives; these stories form a vital counterpoint to the authors' more philosophical thoughts on the subjects of terminal illness, dying, death, and the meaning of life, which is never far from the main current of the book: "We're all, in varying degrees, handicapped by the rubble that litters the inner fields of our hearts." An expansive, richly sympathetic book about the last and least-understood phase of life.

   --Kirkus Reviews

No one escapes the trials and tribulations of life. For me, it was cancer with life-threating complications. Fr. Tom Lynch and Barbara Mariconda have skillfully crafted a guide for walking this harrowing path. The mystery of God's saving power is evident in the well laid out practical tools and touching witness stories. This profound work gives readers the courage, faith, hope, and resolve to walk this journey with loved ones in a meaningful, life-giving way. It's never too late to start – *After the Diagnosis: A Guide for Living* can change everything.

   --Linda Mossorofo, cancer survivor

In a world that misunderstands the mystery of serious sickness, Father Tom Lynch and Barbara Mariconda have masterfully narrated a path that offers healing and hope for anyone who is seriously ill. Through their keen insights, personal stories and spiritual wisdom, *After the Diagnosis: A Guide for Living* provides its readers with all the tools needed to seek personal healing and to understand suffering as a catalyst for a renewed life filled with zeal, purpose and an appreciation of the present moment as a gift. I highly recommend this book for anyone who has received a diagnosis of serious illness and wishes to seek healing and hope. I also commend it to anyone who desires to learn how to live life fully, one day at a time.

   --Most Reverend Frank Caggiano, Bishop, Diocese of Bridgeport

After the Diagnosis is a profoundly affecting book both for the seriously ill person and for the caregiver. After my sister received a terminal diagnosis, I found *After the Diagnosis* to be my guidepost, helping me to hold the difficult conversations around death, providing me a handbook for what to expect both physically and emotionally as my sister weakened, and most importantly, teaching me how to be present to this experience in a way that was life-giving and ultimately, transformative. *After the Diagnosis* is a **must read** for any caregiver who desires to experience the dying process of those they dearly love as a time of deep connection, love and peace. An extraordinary book of insight, practicality and spiritual connection.

   --Anne Dichele, Ph.D., Dean, School of Education, Quinnipiac University

As I pondered the profound and practical wisdom that Barbara and Father Tom laid out for you, Robert Frost's poem *The Road not Taken* came to mind. *After The Diagnosis: A Guide for Living* gives us the choice to rethink all our previous notions about the dying process and shows us how choosing the road less traveled can make a difference in our lives and the lives of our loved ones.

   --Father Carl Arico, Founding Member of Contemplative Outreach, author of *The Gift of Life, Death and Dying* - Life and Living program with Thomas Keating, and author of *A Taste of Silence, Centering Prayer and the Contemplative Journey*

Let *After the Diagnosis: A Guide for Living* unfold for you the beauty and infinite depth of love that can be found in even the most difficult, darkest times in our lives. Father Tom Lynch's and Barbara Mariconda's book is a trusted companion to help us find meaning and value in suffering and loss, the path (not always easy) that God is calling us to accept and share in the totality of His love. At a time when medical treatment can become overwhelming, the wisdom and guidance provided by Fr. Tom and Barbara help us cut through the noise and clutter, to discover our ultimate purpose, and to learn that our most important work still lies ahead.

   --Lenore Snowden-Opalak M.D., Internal Medicine, Compassionate Care Award Recipient

I was recently invited to read Fr. Tom and Barbara's book *After the Diagnosis: A Guide for Living.* Being in good health, with things going well in my life, I wondered what was in it for me. As I read, it became apparent - this book is for *anyone* who wants to enrich and deepen their experience of life - to love more deeply, forgive freely, experience hope and joy, to be at peace with self, and one with God. The more I read, the more I saw its relevance. I have truly been transformed by this book. After reading it, I decided to purchase copies for all those I love - my husband, my children, my friends. And I urge you to do the same.

--Mary Margaret Fiscella, R.N.

Tom Lynch knows a thing or two about death and dying. For over 30 years he has pastored a large urban Catholic parish. He has ministered to count-less individuals and families in the clutch of death or terminal illness. He has learned how to lead them to escape the paralyzing grip of denial and to discover in their own stories traces of the great Christian story of redemption, love and life eternal. In *After the Diagnosis: A Guide for Living* Father Lynch shares the gentle humor and unflinching honesty that have led so many to face the mystery of death with Christian hope and peace. His experience and insights provide a pastoral toolkit for priests and others who minister to the dying.

--Reverend Thomas Boland, Retired Pastor, Former President of National Association of Family Life Ministers, Marriage and Family Counselor, Archdiocese of Louisville, Ky.

Just as we prepare for many events in our lives, we need to prepare for our own final journeys. *After the Diagnosis* provides detailed insights into our faith, and teaches us how to fully embrace our lives *now,* regardless of where we find our-selves. I wish I'd had this book during my years as a caregiver for aging parents, and throughout my career as an emergency room and surgical nurse. It would have given me the tools to better understand what the terminally ill and their loved ones were going through, emotionally and spiritually. The Reverend Thomas F. Lynch and Barbara Mariconda remind us that God is always there for us, waiting with open arms.

--Bridget Pardee, R.N.

Quite by chance I met Fr. Tom Lynch and Barbara Mariconda. A few days later we were sitting in my living room chatting about *After the Diagnosis: A Guide for Living.* After reading the book I put it to immediate use with a friend, now 92, who said to me, "I have lived too long, I am worried and cannot see ahead." Well...that was my opening to talk about Father Tom and Barbara's book. Their advice is dead on right. It is inspirational, practical, pulls no punches, and opens the dialogue without offending beliefs in any religion. We need a wider forum for discussing the challenging issues after receiving a diagnosis – a journey we each are destined to take from the day of our births. This book carries the discussion to new heights and helps the patient and loved ones live life to the fullest while facing the realities of dying and death.

--Gail Matthews, Author of *Did I Die? Managing the Mayhem of Alzheimer's: A Caregiver's Guide to Peace and Quality of Life*

This book is dedicated to all who have walked the
Path of Suffering,
and have taught us well along the way.

Acknowledgments

MANY THANKS TO Fr. Thomas Boland and Fr. Carl Arico, for their persistent encouragement and critical input throughout this process. Also, thanks to Virginia Weir and Anne Dichele for their straight-forward critiques and ongoing support, both literary and spiritual. The authors wish to also thank Fathers Boland and Arico, and Virginia and Anne for the great gift of their friendship. We'd also like to express appreciation to Sr. Kateri Battaglia, Sr. Carol Dempsey, Linda Mossorofo, and Dr. Lenore Snowden Opalak, who graciously served as readers prior to publication. Likewise, this book could not have found its way into print without the untiring work of Marcy Kelly, both in terms of feedback and administrative support. Many thanks to Deidra Golino Lodge for our cover design and logo, and to Josh Dichele of the Dichele Group for reflecting our work on our website. Also, thanks to Mary Plamieniak for sharing her expertise in getting the word out there. Lastly, we are deeply grateful to Bishop Frank Caggiano for his careful reading and support throughout the process.

Your Most Fulfilling Work is Ahead of You...

Rocco, a successful businessman, had lived life in the fast lane, affording himself all the bennies and perks associated with success. At 58, Rocco was diagnosed with pancreatic cancer. He was stunned – the man who'd been able to do it all, a self-proclaimed master of his own destiny, who lived and never looked back, had been stopped in his tracks. He left the doctor's office, shell-shocked and overwhelmed. Now what?

Rocco somehow made it to his car, and without making a conscious decision to do so, found himself driving to his mother's grave. He got out, sat on the ground, put his head in his hands and cried. "Mom," he sobbed, "What am I gonna do? "

He felt his mother's presence in an overwhelming way. This was followed by a strong impulse to somehow "get back to God." Rocco got up, thanked his mother, and came to see me.

Not one to beat around the bush, I told him, "Rocco, you have a challenging path ahead of you. But, your greatest work – the most important and fulfilling work of your life is ahead of you." This began our journey together for the next two years.

Rocco put his hand to the plow and began to approach his faith as he had his work and his play – jumping in with both feet.

He returned to church with some regularity, and actively reached out to make amends for whatever hurt he had caused his loved ones. He also strived to build deeper relationships with family and friends, spending time in conversation as well as companionable silence - for the first time becoming a man of *presence* rather than *presents*. We'd go to breakfast and engage in deep conversations about life, love, and death. Rocco actively shared his spiritual reading and insights with others, and spoke openly about the transformation he was experiencing. He still had a fun-loving personality, went to the casinos, and enjoyed life as best as he could, living as fully as he could right up to the day he died.

Toward the end of Rocco's life I stopped by his house. He invited me to join him in his garage, where he'd go for a smoke. "What the hell? "

he said, exhaling through a smile, savoring the tobacco that could no longer hurt him. He took another drag, looked me in the eye and said, "Fr. Tom, these past two years have been the happiest years of my life. How I wish I knew back then what I know now..."

Several weeks later, on his death-bed, I came to see him again. He asked me to lie down beside him so he could whisper in my ear. "I love you," he murmured, his face lit with a smile of deep joy. He died shortly thereafter, leaving a legacy of transformation and of love. He never lost his zest for living, or his passion in dying.

This is what I want for you, as well.

The Table of Contents

Chapter-by-chapter questions for discussion and reflection can be
found at www.journeyofthesoulbooks.com

Introduction

No doubt, you've picked up this book for one of several reasons. Either you or someone you love is facing a serious or terminal illness. You might be standing in the wake of a death or find yourself dealing with loved ones mired in it. Perhaps you're a professional who has dedicated your life to helping others in this situation. Or, maybe you're one of the few people curious enough about the emotional, spiritual, and physical challenges of sickness, dying, and death to begin the quest long before your own final chapter.

For most of us, facing our own impending death or that of a loved one is the greatest challenge we'll ever be confronted with. We try to control the mystery of it by dealing with it on our own terms - fighting against it, or running from the brokenness of human existence rather than allowing it to reveal any greater meaning.

But, what if it was possible to enter into this process in a free and loving way? To see sickness and death as sacred, to reverence the great mystery of it? What if we could avoid the paralyzing fear, denial, anger, and regret that so often colors what could be a life-giving, redemptive, and liberating experience? And, ultimately, during this often elongated process, what if we could live fully even as we're dying, in a gracious and loving way?

That is what this book is all about.

We want to engage you in a new conversation about sickness, suffering, and dying. Instead of viewing the movement as a "winding down" of life, we can begin to recognize it as a natural thrust toward wholeness, rooted in our oneness with all that is, was, and will be. The entire continuum can be seen as our evolution toward a higher level of consciousness, empowering us to experience the eternal quality that we share with the universe and everything in it. This book is intended to gently guide you toward a deep knowing that death is not the end, that it doesn't have to destroy the bonds we've forged in our lives, and that love doesn't stop at the grave.

Of course, completing what we think of as the final leg of our earthly journey poses a number of challenging transitions. Most of us will move through a period of denial, then resignation, and for some, on to a state of acceptance. Much has been written about acceptance – many books and programs are designed to take you there.

But this book is different.

Instead, we want to share a rare slice of heaven that can be grasped on *this* side of the grave. A place beyond acceptance, and before death. A place of transformation in which we can realize what our life's purpose has been, and what an amazing gift we can entrust to those we leave behind. How our legacy can be one of love – pure, powerful, and eternal.

So, this book is not just about sickness, dying, and death – it's about rebirth *in this life and beyond*. It's really about living and loving along the *entire* journey. **Most importantly, the realization that we can *choose* the way we live and the way we *love* through every stage of living, sickness, dying, and death can change *everything*.**

During my 30 years as pastor of a large Catholic parish I've officiated at over 1,500 funerals. I've watched families struggle, fight, and throw away what could be a precious shared time together. I've also seen the opposite – loved ones who walk together down this mysterious pathway in a shared sense of intimacy, awe, appreciation, and love, leading to a profound awareness of the gift of the other and the presence and power of God. They've been able to *transform* the starkness and suffering inherent along the pathway toward death.

The *transformative power of love* is what makes all the difference. When we begin the process of moving away from our "ego selves" toward our true "spirit selves," when we learn to embrace mystery rather than our compulsion to control, we gradually grow into the spiritual beings we were always meant to be – and always *have* been, if only we'd been able to recognize it. In doing so we can escape the oppressive anxiety and self-absorption that can dominate our final time on this earth, and instead deepen our awareness of what is at the core of all life - love. Unconditional love. Connectedness. Communion. A wholly fulfilling sense of being one with those we love, with the world, and with all of creation. We begin to experience the indwelling of God, to make meaning of our suffering, to see the purpose of life. To leave behind a legacy of faith, hope, and love.

The depth of your faith experience doesn't matter. Nor does your religious affiliation. Regardless of spiritual practice or lack of it we are all, at the center of our being, one with God. The common path through sickness, dying, and death is an opportunity to explore the indwelling of God, and in the process, discover how to transform our own experience and that of those we care for in and through God's love. While this book is written through the lens of the Catholic Christian faith, the ideas, insights, and practices point to universal core truths that make them applicable to all religious traditions.

You'll find this book to be reflective, but also extremely practical. We offer concrete suggestions and strategies for patients, loved ones, and caregivers. We share stories of the scores of families and individuals who have honored me by allowing me to walk with them on what is always a deeply intimate and personal journey. We invite you to learn from them. Their stories will make you realize that you're not alone.

HOW TO USE THIS BOOK

The best time to approach this material is in the "green times" - the earlier in the process the better. The longer you wait, the more difficult it is to do the real work of living – and of dying. So often families wait far too long to address what's happening, to have the open, honest, and loving conversations that cement the bonds of love and family.

Once you begin you can move through the book in a number of ways. You might sit down and swallow it up whole, then go back and access the sections that best speak to you at each step of your journey. Or, you might pick it up and move through it slowly, savoring it, getting your heart around it a little at a time, like an acquired taste.

After each chapter we encourage you to discuss what you've read with others. On our website (www.journeyofthesoulbooks.com) you'll find discussion questions – food for thought that will help you relate the chapter material to your situation. Since this isn't a "one-and-done" kind of book, I recommend going back to these questions and notes at a later date to contemplate how your perspective may have changed.

So, let the sacred surrender begin – and in the process allow yourself and those you care for to become empowered and healed by love itself.

The Path of Suffering

CHAPTER 1

Life Turns on a Dime

LIFE TURNS ON a dime.

Your boss says, "I'm sorry, we have to let you go."

You read the email – from your husband's lover.

A police officer arrives at your door – there's been a terrible accident.

The emergency room calls – your son overdosed.

The biopsy is positive.

The doctor tells you, "I'm sorry…it's terminal…"

The list goes on and on. Every example involves some kind of an ending, a loss, a *death*.

If you've lived even a little, you've heard these kinds of stories. If you haven't experienced any of them personally, without a doubt, someday you will. In fact, any and all loss we experience in our lives is a precursor to and a rehearsal for death. And death is the greatest loss of all.

Life by its very nature involves suffering. It has the potential to hurt us, to take away everything we hold near and dear. We're all vulnerable to the tremendous pain living can cause. We recognize this as we witness the suffering of others, or walk behind the coffins of those we know. While we feel great sympathy for them, sympathy's shadow side is often relief. Relief that catastrophe has once again passed us by.

Though we often deny it, we know, that eventually, we all will die. It's easy to imagine a far-off death at the end of our golden years, the edges of that vision, blurred, hazy, and comfortably distant. But, the reality is, death takes no prisoners. It strikes where, when, and how it wants. We do everything we can to avoid receiving its inevitable calling card: *It's your turn to die.*

3

Intellectually, we know that death is a natural part of the cycle of life. In our birth we carry the seeds of death, but also of rebirth. This is, in fact, the blueprint for every living thing – trees, plants, flowers, the galaxies and the stars – all of creation.

But, if death is such a natural part of life, why is it that when we, or someone we love winds up holding death's calling card, it brings us to our knees? The person suffering and everyone around them becomes so frightened, angry, and/or full of anxiety that even a conversation about death is a challenge.

GETTING REAL ABOUT DEATH

Early on in my priesthood, before the chrism oil was even dry on my hands, I learned a life-changing lesson about the sometimes un-nameable needs of those with terminal illnesses. And it has shaped every meaningful encounter with the dying and their families that I've had in my 47 years of ministry.

It was my first assignment and the pastor sent me to visit an elderly parishioner named Chester, who had very little time left. I approached the run-down house and rang the bell. I heard someone shuffling to the door – it took a good while before a crusty, stooped old man with several days worth of stubble on his face opened the door. Chester sighed when he saw me, turned, and barked, "Come in. Sit."

I followed him into the dank-smelling room. The shades were drawn and the place was cluttered and dirty. The air was stale, heavy. He dropped into a chair and waved his thin hand, indicating where I was to sit.

Before I had a chance to introduce myself, Chester pointed at me and glared beneath bushy brows.

"Listen, Priest," he said. "If you've come here to give me any of your pious crap, don't waste your breath. Just get back up and find your way to the door. See, here's how it is – when *you're* sick, you know you're going to feel lousy for a few days or even a week. Then you're gonna get better. But me? Every day I feel sick, and the next day I'm even sicker. And I know there won't be a single morning when I get up stronger than I was the day before. It will just get worse and worse 'til the day I finally die."

As I groped for some meaningful way to respond, Chester continued. "And don't tell me to pray – I've prayed day and night, and for what? " He swept his hand across the room, at the array of medical paraphernalia littering every surface, the portable invalid toilet and hospital bed, the collection of pill bottles, the walker. "Didn't your Bible say, ask and ye shall receive? " He snorted. "So, don't bullshit me. Be real. Or get the hell out of here."

I knew the scripture Chester was referring to – the book of Matthew, chapter 7:

> *"Ask and it will be given to you; seek and you will find; knock and the door will be opened to you. For anyone who asks, receives; and the one who seeks finds, to the one who knocks, the door will be opened."*

I thought about explaining that God's will is inscrutable, and that suffering can be redemptive. These were things we discussed in the seminary. But, looking at Chester, I knew that response would be met with disdain. And, if truth be told, it felt hugely inadequate.

But I realized something. Chester had let me in. He offered me that much confidence – or maybe it was hope. Clearly, he wanted *something* from me. It wasn't theology. It wasn't sympathy or false optimism. And it wasn't formal, impersonal prayer. He'd resigned himself to his situation, and was desperately trying to find meaning in it. He needed to know where God was in all of it. His life had turned on a dime – his diagnosis - the turning point, the defining moment that divided his life into *before* and *after.* The person he had once been was gone. There had to be a way to redefine himself – but there was no way to go back and reclaim who he'd been, seemingly no way to go forward, and no one to guide him.

At the time, I had little to offer. I asked him to tell me about his illness, which he did. I listened in awkward silence. Finally, I asked if I could anoint him. He agreed, and grateful for something to do, I read the prayers and performed the ritual – hiding behind the words and prescribed movements. He grudgingly accepted this and afterward I wished him well, told him I'd keep him in prayer and made my exit. I felt his eyes following me out the door. Moving along the front walk I knew I'd let him down and left him unfulfilled. That feeling of having missed the mark stayed with me a long time. Chester died shortly afterward, but I continued to reflect on our exchange. He had somehow invited me to holy ground – the place where God was working - but at the time I just didn't have the insight or ability to go there.

I later realized that what he was asking for, in his own gruff way, was for someone to be able to walk in his shoes for a little while, to *understand* what his difficult journey was like. He desperately needed to talk about what death meant. He longed for someone who would *listen,* for someone who had the courage to honor his experience and emotions with an honest response. But most of all he needed the insight and wisdom that would allow him to make meaning not only of his suffering, but of the life that was drawing to a close. Chester was seeking something that would empower him to put his experience in a greater context. To transform his suffering and make him know that, somehow, his life and what he was experiencing *mattered.* Chester needed a loving guide to walk with him along the path on which he was embarking. There he was, facing the most frightening, mysterious, and important event of his life and there was no one to validate it, to point the way, to help him transform his suffering into something deeply relevant. Imagine what a haunted, lonely place that must have been.

OUR INABILITY TO DEAL WITH DEATH

Our inability to deal with death can paralyze us, robbing us of peace in whatever days we, or a loved one, have remaining. Our culture's taboo in this regard often forces us, before we die, into a grave of our own making. It demonizes a natural process and refuses to recognize any value in suffering. By not acknowledging and dealing with the reality of sickness and an impending death, negative emotions intensify – fear, anger, anxiety, loneliness, bitterness, guilt, resentment, ambivalence.

Unresolved issues, unmet expectations, and complicated family dynamics become magnified, fueled by our insistence on trying to control the uncontrollable.

All of this begs the question: **Does it have to be this way?** How can we overcome these obstacles to freedom so that we, or a loved one, can die in a spirit of peace and hopeful joy, open to the transformative mystery about to be revealed that not only radically changes our lives but the lives of those who journey with us?

THE ESSENTIAL QUESTION

One of the most natural and at the same time most challenging questions children ask is this: *What happens to us when we die?*

Our response, geared to the young, is meant to offer solace in a simple, straight-forward way. We say, *When we die we go to heaven.* Or, *grandma is up in heaven looking down on us.*

These explanations might temporarily satisfy an eight-year-old, but do little to assuage the fears of adults as they face the biggest transition in their lives. Those of us who hold some kind of traditional religious beliefs usually acknowledge, in an abstract or a theological way, that there's something more than life here and now. Catholics and other Christians profess this, *"I believe in the resurrection of the dead and the life of the world to come, the resurrection of the body, and life eternal."*

Somehow, though we recite the words, when we receive a serious diagnosis, they don't seem to resonate, because as adults, that question – *What will happen to me when I die* - begs a greater response. It was surely one question that had haunted Chester.

If I'd met Chester today, after nearly 50 years of walking this path with the sick, the dying, their families and caregivers, I'd be able to offer a larger picture. At their most vulnerable, these parishioners, family members, and friends have taught me much. They forced me to grow up, they've strengthened my faith, they've opened my eyes.

Fortunately, what I didn't know then, I can share with you, now. As an entré into the conversation, I would have acknowledged the many ways

Chester's world was shrinking. I would have validated his feelings, his sense of loss, his fear, his anger and grief at what was being taken from him. I would have assured him that what he was feeling was exactly what we all will feel at some point - because we're human. And then, more importantly, I would have gently asked Chester to imagine a larger reality than the ever-diminishing stage of his life. To recognize the subtle evidence of a much bigger story, an expanded script, in which this life that we know is only Act One. As Chester's sense of autonomy was being threatened, as his capacities were being stripped from him, and as the man he prided himself on being began to seem like a faded memory, I would have told him that his most important work was ahead of him. That, if he would consent to it, he could tap into a power so much greater than himself. A power that could change the texture of this difficult journey - not only for himself, but for those he loved.

Chester, I know, would have challenged me. But I would have his attention. I'd be real with him. I'd talk with him about the road ahead, without pulling any punches.

And that is why I've written this book. So that I can have this conversation with you.

So, back to the original question – what happens when we die?

Maybe a better place to start is with a couple of different, but parallel questions – what is the trajectory of human life? Is death the end, or is it a doorway?

I'd like to sketch out a kind of roadmap that I call "The Journey of the Soul." This roadmap is focused on the work of God in our lives, yesterday, today, and tomorrow.

But, before I do, keep in mind that whenever we aspire to see beyond our own myopic view of life, we enter the realm of mystery. Mystery, by its very nature, isn't meant to be deconstructed or analyzed. Instead, mystery is to be embraced, marveled over, and approached with a sense of awe and hope. In talking about mystery we're limited by our human experience and by the constraints of language. It isn't literal, but figurative. It's more poetic than pragmatic. I invite you to open yourself, through eyes of faith, to the mystery that Scripture points to, that religious traditions have forever sought to profess, embrace, and celebrate.

THE JOURNEY OF THE SOUL

Our life here on earth is just the first of three phases of living – only one portion of a journey that begins and ends with God. This journey of the soul is grounded in the following truth that we know only partially, especially in this earthly phase of the process: *that we're completely one with God, unconditionally loved by God, and one with all that is.*

I wish I'd told Chester that he was standing in a uniquely sacred place where he could experience a powerful sense of this wholeness, of communion, of an intimate, vital link to God. I'd have explained to Chester that there's a "generative thrust" of the spirit that would carry him through the entire journey.

Unfortunately, at the time, I hadn't the experience or maturity of faith to talk to Chester about the Journey of the Soul.

But, now I do. After years of studying the Scriptures in the context of the Catholic Church's tradition, walking this path with so many, and having my faith seasoned by the realities of life, I've found the following imagery helpful.

Think of an escalator that carries us from the moment of birth to eternity. Let's take a ride on this escalator through the three phases of the Journey of the Soul.

FIRST PHASE OF LIVING: A SPIRIT IN GOD – BIRTH – LIFE – DYING

Even before our birth, each of us existed as a spirit in God. When we're born into this world, this spirit of God continues to dwell within us. Though we're largely unaware of it, there's a "generative thrust," a deep longing inside us that continually draws us toward wholeness and a sense of oneness with God and all God's creation. We're born with the gifts of God's unconditional love, mercy, forgiveness, and healing. If we open ourselves to these gifts, if we explore and nurture them, we recognize that the question God is always asking is this: *Will you let me love you?*

Unfortunately, as we grow and become members of the culture, we often lose touch with this core spirit of God that gives us life. We grow into adulthood, establish ourselves, build our ego strengths. At the same time, life wounds us. People let us down, we experience every kind of loss. Often, we hurt ourselves. Through it all, our God waits, eager for us to open the gifts we have inside, asking again: *Will you let me love you?*

The degree to which we recognize the indwelling of God and cooperate with the life-giving thrust also changes the texture of how we deal with every aspect of life. The rest of this book explores the earthly portion of the escalator ride – how we can cooperate with God's generative thrust, and how we can respond to God's ongoing overture of love.

Regardless of the extent to which we respond to God, death allows not only the complete release of our bodies and of all of our human concerns - it also releases the self-induced restrictions on the God-given gifts that we've had inside us all along. Death is the doorway that brings us to Phase Two...

SECOND PHASE OF LIVING: RESURRECTION OF THE DEAD – PURIFICATION – ONENESS WITH GOD

At the moment of death, we emerge from the darkness and travel toward a great light – the living and loving presence of God. We call this "the resurrection of the dead." This departure of the life force, the energy, the very essence and soul leaves the body inert and empty. Though the body is present, we say things like "He's gone," or "She's passed." What moves on to this second phase is the heart and the soul, carrying with them any unhealed wounds and sins. But that's not all. We also carry with us God's gifts of unconditional love, mercy, forgiveness, and healing. These gifts had been given to us at birth, but the challenges of the first phase of living often prevent us from being open to them. But, in phase two we have the opportunity to experience God's gifts in a greater way.

Sometimes people worry. They say to me, "But Fr. Tom, I wasn't much of a church-goer." Even for those who had little interest in their faith during most of the first phase, when seeing their God face-to-face, have the opportunity to say "yes" to God's question: *Will you let me love you?* They can finally open their hearts to a loving encounter with their God. When I explained this to one family, the wife, who was just a month away from death said to me, "Fr. Tom, this *is* good news! It gives me tremendous hope."

Of course, some may choose not to say yes to God, intentionally extending the isolation they established during Phase One – and we call that separation *hell*. The choice is always ours. I tell families that this is why it's important to pray for the dead – to pray that they may finally say yes to God's open invitation, to surrender to God's love. When this happens the deceased will be able to love those left behind as God loves them – unconditionally.

The wounds of the heart are very much entwined with the spirit self, and during the process of purification (sometimes referred to as purgation) the spirit fully opens to God's compassionate love (which we call God's mercy). This involves the cleansing of any sin that remains, and the healing of any stories or wounds that, during life, prevented us from letting ourselves be loved by God and others. We experience God's forgiveness so that we can, at last, forgive whoever or whatever placed these wounds on our hearts during the first phase of living. In other words, hanging onto un-forgiveness prevents the wounds of our hearts from being healed by divine love. When we allow ourselves to be unconditionally forgiven and healed we can finally and fully enter into oneness with God – our hearts becoming one with God's heart.

In Phase Two we continue this movement toward "wholeness" in a deeper way, and realize our true, undefended selves in God. We embrace this new oneness with God and all that is - Where God is - that is where we are: in all of creation, in every person we left behind, as well as all who ever lived (Catholics call this the Communion of Saints). Pope Francis affirms this powerful reality: "There is a deep and indissoluble bond between those who are still pilgrims in this world -– us – and those who have crossed the threshold of death and entered eternity." I tell families, "When your loved one dies, the rest of you will be left behind in the first phase of living. But when you access the God within, you'll also touch into the love of the deceased." In this oneness with God the deceased also shares in God's longing, *"Will you let me love you?"* Unlike human love, their love for you is now pure and unconditional. This love doesn't present itself as a dramatic apparition or message from beyond. Instead, you will be presented with gentle promptings of the spirit that encourage you to respond to God's presence within you. Experiencing a greater ability to love, to forgive, to serve others – these are the fruits of this divine union.

THIRD PHASE OF LIVING: RESURRECTION OF THE BODY – LIFE ETERNAL

At the end of all time, at the close of the world as we know it (the last days), we will be birthed again into a glorified body to embrace life eternal, in love with our God and with all that is. This is the promise, the covenant between God and humankind, revealed in the death and resurrection of Jesus Christ. In the Book of Revelation (Chapter 21) God promised us "new heavens and a new earth." But what this will look like remains a mystery.

But what we do know is this – after his death Jesus appeared to his disciples as a living and loving presence, but they had a hard time recognizing him in this new form. The Gospels tell us that Mary Magdalene mistook him for the gardener at the empty tomb, and his disciples failed to recognize him along the road to Emmaus. In his reappearance Jesus demonstrated that there's life after death, and that we'll be birthed again in a new form (a glorified body.) This is reflected both in scripture and in ritual. In John 6:39-40 Jesus says, *"And this is the will of the one who sent me, that I should not lose anything of what he gave me, but that I should raise it on the last day."*

(Will you let me love you?)

Likewise, in the funeral rite of the church, at the committal, the presider prays: "The Lord Jesus Christ will change our mortal bodies to be like his in glory, for he is risen, the firstborn from the dead. So let us commend our brother/sister to the Lord that the Lord may embrace him/her in peace and raise up his/her body on the last day." *(Will you let me love you?)*

To be human is to be embodied. At our birth, in the first phase, we're born in flesh and blood, and the promise is that we'll be enfleshed again in the third phase. Jesus showed us this when he returned to his disciples, emphasizing that "it is real," insisting that they touch him, speak with him, share a meal together. He wanted them to understand that just as he lived among them in the first phase, so he would live among them again, in a new glorified form. This is our hope as we journey toward the end of our earthly existence. It's what we proclaim in our creed and celebrate in the Eucharist. It's just that we tend to look at it theologically and intellectually, with little pause for the ramifications of what Jesus sought to show us.

This is where the escalator stops, at life eternal. It means we're going to be in love with God, in love with one another, forever. This is our destiny and purpose, at the end of all time.

That is the Good News.

Unfortunately, as most of us begin to traverse the Path of Suffering inherent in the dying process, we fail to see it.

My Lord God,
I have no idea where I am going.
I do not see the road ahead of me.
I cannot know for certain where it will end.
Nor do I really know myself, and the fact that I think I am
following Your Will does not mean that I am actually doing so.
But I believe that the desire to please You does in fact please You.
And I hope I have that desire in all that I am doing.
I hope that I will never do anything apart from that desire.
And I know that if I do this, you will lead me by the right road,
though I may know nothing about it.
Therefore, I will trust You always though I may seem
to be lost and in the shadow of death.
I will not fear, for You are ever with me, and
You will never leave me to face my perils alone.

THOMAS MERTON - *THOUGHTS IN SOLITUDE*
ABBEY OF GETHSEMANI

CHAPTER 2

Walking the Path of Suffering

MY EXPERIENCE WITH Chester profoundly affected me. And my vocation continued to present one situation after another that reiterated the question: *Does it have to be this way?* The issue became even more pressing, not only in terms of what I could offer as I attempted to minister to people in need, but in regard to the faith I was ordained to preach.

I realized that in order to minister in a meaningful way to the sick and dying, I'd need to enter into and really strive to understand their world. So, I took every opportunity to spend time, talk, and be real with them. I asked them to help me articulate what they were going through. In listening empathetically I began to recognize a predictable series of challenges inherent in the process. As I walked with parishioners, family members, and friends, this Path of Suffering became more and more familiar to me. It was a journey replete with hazards along the way – the road, rough, with deep ditches on either side. This path led through a dark wilderness, through territory few cared to explore. And, the sick and the dying weren't the only travelers I met on this road. Often caretakers of the chronically, seriously, or terminally ill find themselves along this route, sometimes becoming the silent victims of the person they're caring for – recipients of displaced anger, regret, and bitterness. The caregiver's suffering often goes unrecognized, as it is overshadowed by the more obvious suffering of the loved one in their care. Still others struggled with a variety of losses - a home in foreclosure, a divorce or shattering of any significant relationship, the death of a dream – they also found themselves wandering on the path. While the specific circumstances and degrees of suffering varied, the basic roadmap remained the same.

I continue to see, first-hand, how the landscape of the path often produces physical discomfort or pain, and with it, emotional distress, mental anguish, and even spiritual darkness. The journey requires all of these reluctant pilgrims to relinquish control, to let go of things they'd prefer to hold on to. The stripping away produces a myriad of powerful feelings – fear, anxiety, sadness, anger, regret, grief, isolation, self-absorption - the intensity of these feelings commensurate with the seriousness of the impending loss.

In the past, a terminal diagnosis usually meant imminent death. But today the process that begins with a sobering diagnosis continues with a series of treatments that can prolong life for an extended number of years. So, depending on the nature of the situation, the Path of Suffering may be punctuated by periods of relative calm. Patients might experience a temporary respite or their disease might go into remission. So, learning to live gracefully while dying, or how to traverse the various stages of the path is more important now than ever before. This kind of a temporary reprieve provides a great opportunity to begin to face the reality and use the time well.

In the case of someone swept from life in an instant, for example, from a heart attack or car accident – in their absence their loved ones are thrust onto this way of suffering. Those diminished by Alzheimer's or dementia may not be cognizant of the path they're on, but family and friends bear the cross for them.

Regardless of the circumstances, at some point, *all* of us will have to take this journey, either as patient, caregiver, or a victim of the harshness of life.

So, I had to ask myself, is there any reason for hope? Is our life simply ticking away, second by second, bringing us closer to this inevitable Path of Suffering? And if so, is there any redemptive value in it? *And, perhaps, most importantly – if the path is inevitable, does the way we decide to take this walk matter? Can we determine what our stance will be in the face of these difficulties?*

After so many years of guiding people along this course, the answer is a resounding *yes*, we *can* choose the manner in which we respond to the significant challenges inherent in the journey. The stance we take can radically transform the experience for ourselves and for those who travel with us.

I'm *not* talking about making lemonade out of lemons. Nor am I here to be a cheerleader plugging the false optimism typified by urging you to "look on the bright side." That would discredit and disrespect the depth and breadth of your experience. What I want for you is so much more than that.

THE LAY OF THE LAND

It's important to take a closer look at the emotions associated with the incremental losses typically experienced along the way. If you're a caregiver, this chapter will help you better understand what the patient is going through. It will also validate the often unacknowledged suffering that you're experiencing as well. If you're the one dealing with a serious or terminal illness you'll benefit by having a roadmap. No one wants to begin an arduous trek without a travel guide. It will also help you to see that your loved ones are on the path alongside you, thus allowing you to better help one another. Together on this path, it is possible to form a "soul partnership" (Chapter 23) that can transform the journey for both of you into one characterized by unconditional love. Whether caregiver or patient, knowing what to expect can help you prepare to confront what lies ahead. Anticipating and then recognizing the signposts along the road will validate and honor your own experience or that of a loved one. While no two journeys are alike, you can be assured that what you're feeling is in some way what we all have experienced or *will* experience, and that, in fact, you're not alone.

Seeing the stark reality of the path is the first step toward transformation – and the rest of this book is dedicated to that.

Signposts along the Path of Suffering – Where do you find yourself?

Recently I met with a parishioner who's struggled with an inoperable brain tumor for almost two years. "Father Tom," she said. "No one understands what this is *like!*" I could feel the intensity of her pain, and her sense of isolation in it. I took out a piece of paper and said, "Maria, you're not alone. What you're experiencing is normal along this Path of Suffering." Then I drew out the following chart and asked her to have a look at it and add her personal experience to whatever signposts spoke to her.

The Path of Suffering

1. **Dealing with Overwhelming Thoughts and Emotions**
2. **Relying on Your Instinctive Coping Mechanisms**
3. **Interacting with Family and Friends**
4. **Navigating Outside Support Systems**
5. **Grappling with Your Faith**
6. **Feeling Tired, Stuck, and Relationally Depleted**
7. **Realizing there's No Turning Back**
8. **Traversing the Dark Hole**
9. **Adapting to a New Normal**
10. **Who am I Becoming?**

"Yes!" she said, suddenly animated. "I've experienced *all* of these signposts."

Then Maria and I discussed each of them.

As you read each signpost, don't despair – the rest of the book will outline a new way of approaching this predictable path. We'll give you the tools – the knowledge, the insight, the faith and hope necessary to dispel your fear and allow you to live in a radical joy until the day death touches you. But, for now, facing the reality of the path, un-sugar-coated, can help you to commit to another way of being.

1. SIGNPOST: DEALING WITH OVERWHELMING EMOTIONS

A difficult situation or a tragedy has landed right in your lap. When your life turns on a dime, it reveals the brokenness of human existence, how unfair it can be. When Larry lost his two daughters (his only two children) in a car crash he was shocked, shaken to the core. The situation seemed surreal, his life suddenly felt as if it was moving in slow motion. His psychological and spiritual suffering was intense. He was overcome by strong emotions – rage, debilitating sadness, tremendous fear. Other times he just felt numb.

When thrust into a situation like Larry's, at some point the numbness begins to wear off, and you can't believe that life has dealt you such an unfair hand. "Why me? " is a question you'll likely ask, over and over again. "Why has God allowed this to happen? " Obsessively asking these unanswerable questions produces even greater mental anguish. You feel constantly bullied by repetitive, unrelenting thoughts. These thoughts kick up powerful emotions that become increasingly inflamed. All of this moves you into the future where fears and anxieties ambush you. Tears are close to the surface, but you hold them back because you have the sense that if you allow yourself to cry you may never regain control.

2. SIGNPOST: RELYING ON YOUR INSTINCTIVE COPING MECHANISMS

You're torn between the desire to crawl up in a ball and retreat, or to be strong and fight with everything you've got. Raging thoughts and emotions can activate a state of denial, providing some space in which to adjust and cope. At first you may avoid dealing with the situation, out of an instinctive sense of self-protection. In the case of a terminal diagnosis, in which your very life is threatened, there's a natural thrust toward survival at all cost. Eventually you may become resigned to the situation and focus all of your attention on trying to control the uncontrollable. This single-hearted attention on treatment, on fighting the symptoms, prevents you from reflecting on the deeper implications of the disease in regard to relationships and the quality and meaning of life. These natural coping mechanisms (denial, resignation and acceptance) will automatically become your modus operandi as you encounter each of the following signposts along this path. If you don't *intentionally* choose another way to respond, you'll live each day in a radically self-absorbed stance, coping and controlling, giving away whatever time you have left. (More on these natural coping mechanisms in Chapters 5-8.)

3. SIGNPOST: INTERACTING WITH FAMILY AND FRIENDS

Your illness will require a redefinition of family roles and rules. It will demand that you all renegotiate who does what, when, and how. How open or closed is your family system? How close or separate will the family members be? How flexible or structured is your "new normal"? The answers to these questions can cause relief, confusion, or resentment. As I always say, "Where two or three are gathered in the family's name, let the games begin!" You may not want to relinquish control of your duties, and others may not want to take them on. And yet, in order to adapt to the demands of the illness, change is inevitable. Often when family members try to help, it's difficult to let them love and care for you. Some of them over-function and drive you crazy. You feel suffocated by their constant worry and attention. Others may under-function, making you wonder if they expect you to shoulder this alone. If they haven't yet dealt with their own vulnerability, losses, or mortality they'll either be in your face, or withdraw – seeing you struggling with the very thing they're most threatened by is just too difficult. Those who've stood in a similar situation will relate to you best, bringing a quiet, empathetic presence.

Whatever their response, allowing loved ones to care for you requires that you acknowledge your own vulnerability, which might frighten or even anger you. You may push them away because you're unwilling to give up whatever control you still have. It's easy to resent the fact that their lives are moving forward, seemingly unencumbered, while yours is stuck. At a time when life is becoming less and less manageable, you'll tend to cling to anything and everything that can make you feel more like your former self. You want to be independent. You want to believe you can do this on your own.

You also might worry, that on some level, these people who profess to love you might actually let you down, because they fail to deliver what you need. This hurls you into a sense of desolation, maybe even anger. When you refuse to let yourself be loved and cared for by those you care about, you risk falling into even greater self-absorption. If this happens, even the most well-intentioned relatives and friends can become the silent victims of your pain and/or emotional suffering due to displaced resentment, fear, anger and sense of loss.

Also, by letting others love and care for you, you risk seeing the fear in their eyes, doubling the sadness you already feel. Often, because of this, those involved become encumbered by an unwritten "code of silence" that prevents honest conversation about the situation. Instead of discussing the complexity of feelings, the conversation focuses on the practicality of treatment, creating a mutually protective façade of false optimism. Without open, honest, and loving conversations that acknowledge the reality of what is, confusion is a given. (More on family dynamics in Chapter 6.)

4. SIGNPOST: NAVIGATING OUTSIDE SUPPORT SYSTEMS

Out of necessity, you turn to professionals and institutions for help. When Grace was diagnosed with breast cancer it seemed her life became an endless stream of doctor's appointments and tests. Her attitude in dealing with medical and other service providers ran the gamut between disdain and adulation. With their sometimes objective, dispassionate demeanor, Grace bounced between feeling like a helpless victim at their mercy, a resistant agitator, or a demanding complainer. She was both beholden to and angry with them. After all, it seemed as though her life was being held rather casually in their hands. They possessed the knowledge, power, and skills she didn't have and desperately needed. Negotiating the line between being her own best advocate and undermining her care by annoying specialists and other caregivers was a constant source of stress. Should she get a second opinion? A third opinion? And, how to get all of her medical professionals on the same page? Should she bring along a family member or friend to listen more objectively? The time between appointments and the endless waiting for test results was a torture for Grace. Her sense of urgency seemed lost on them. She found herself continually asking, "Do any of them really understand what I'm going through? Or am I just one more patient? "

Fortunately many of her professional caregivers extended compassion and empathy along with their medical ministrations. She also recognized that they were more objective than family, in many ways better prepared for guiding her through this uncharted course. At times, however, Grace found herself shifting all her faith to them, in essence, lifting them up as god and savior. Throughout the course of her illness, many options of care were presented to her. Taking responsibility for these decisions was, at times, excruciating. What constituted extraordinary means? What might put a burden on the family? Would the treatment actually relieve her pain or just extend her suffering? This became an emotional roller coaster – her outlook soaring at good news, and crashing when things didn't turn out as hoped. She began to listen selectively, latching onto words of optimism and ignoring others.

5. SIGNPOST: GRAPPLING WITH YOUR FAITH

Most, as they continue to search for answers and seek support, will turn to God. You'll wonder, "Where is God in this? How could God allow this to happen? " You may feel deserted and angry at God. Where is the faith you thought you had? Suffering can be like piling too many logs on the fire of your faith. The flame turns to smoke, and unless the flame is fanned, it can go out.

You might reach out to persons of faith and/or a church or religious community, hoping they'll pray for you and reassure you that God is with you during this difficult time. By its very nature, a community of faith should help us embrace our vulnerability, our losses, and our own mortality.

You might find, however, that the depth of spiritual care you need isn't offered, due to the fact that those ministering to you have not had their own faith tested, or experienced what you're going through. Platitudes don't serve, and doubling down on the prayers and rituals of naïve faith also don't provide the solace and solutions we seek.

When Laura was diagnosed with pancreatic cancer she approached a neighbor who was a devout Catholic. Surely, this woman, who attended daily mass, prayed the rosary, and offered novenas, could ensure a cure. After all, miracles can happen if we believe deeply enough, can't they? As the disease progressed in spite of her neighbor's spiritual intervention, Laura became cynical, angry with God and disillusioned with religion. You might react as Laura did, or you might push away those with strong faith because it raises a mirror to your own, and you feel you'll come up wanting. It's easy to resent others' faith, as it may seem as though God has granted them a grace that you don't have. This can be depressing, because God might appear to be the last resort, and even God isn't delivering.

Consciously or unconsciously, you're struggling with what your religious beliefs and teachings mean, practically, in your situation. You wonder:

- Does my faith empower me to live *and* to die well?
- Does my faith help me to access the living and loving God within me?
- Do my religious beliefs provide me with hope when I have to stand in darkness?
- Does my faith tradition help calm my fears and anxieties when they're inflamed?
- Does my religion provide a sense of peace – that inner stillness that allows me to respond to life in a loving way versus reacting against it?

- Do my religious beliefs and practices help me to stand in and make meaning of suffering?
- Does my religion help me to see my situation in the context of a much larger story?

If the answer to any of these is no, you may be questioning the value of religion – what good is it, anyway? It may feel as though still another system has failed you. If you haven't consistently explored and lived your faith, the answer to these questions will invariably be "no." (In Chapters 7 and 15 we'll look at religion from a much deeper perspective.)

6. SIGNPOST: FEELING TIRED, STUCK, AND RELATIONALLY DEPLETED

Walking this Path of Suffering demands every ounce of your emotional, spiritual, and physical energy, day in and day out. All your attention is focused on trying to turn the situation around. It is all-encompassing, and exhausting.

When Joe began dialysis, life as he knew it changed dramatically. While being tethered to a machine, waiting for the right kidney donor, he had a vein collapse, and contracted a blood infection. He felt physically ill and concern over the changes in his body monopolized his mind. His thoughts raced out of control and worries raged inside him. It was hard to follow a conversation or to engage with anyone in a mindful way. It was as though he was constantly pummeled by negative emotions – there was no way to escape. Throughout the day Joe felt exhausted and his restless nights seemed endless. As soon as the lights went out, the house grew quiet, and he heard his wife's gentle breathing in the dark beside him, all of his worry and anxiety would ambush him. He'd toss and turn until morning when the whole process began again. The days wore on and Joe became more and more stuck – a feeling of being trapped in the situation with no way to escape. The path ahead seemed overwhelming. As his health deteriorated the chances of qualifying for a transplant dimmed. How long is this going to drag on, Joe wondered.

He desperately hoped to get better, but his anger, frustration, and sadness overshadowed his hope. He was tired of the whole thing. Joe's wife felt just as weary – she was often wracked with guilt because, despite her best efforts, she could never seem to do anything to ease his distress. At times she resented that he just couldn't appreciate the fact that she was suffering as well.

Joe and his wife were both sick and tired of dealing with his illness, with doctors, tests, appointments, the stress of shifting family dynamics. They both felt stuck and neither wanted to talk about it. This capped frustration and debilitating fatigue produced anger and depression.

In addition to this, dealing with Joe's sickness left them emotionally and relationally depleted. They were running on empty. It was easier to avoid other people than to have to work at relating to them. Their world continued to shrink. The illness upstaged and overshadowed every other aspect of their lives. They wondered how their relationship had become lost in the disease. They seemed to have nothing left to give.

7. SIGNPOST: REALIZING THERE'S NO TURNING BACK

You want to go back to when life was "normal," you fantasize about what it would be like to somehow miraculously turn things around, but there's a growing realization that you can't. You experience sadness and grief over the loss of what has been. This grief, on top of the depression, sadness, and anger brings about a heaviness that weighs you down.

Some friends may begin to avoid you. Others may try to engage you in meaningless chatter, to distract you, or to pretend that everything will be fine.

When Bill was in the hospital with lung cancer, visitors seemed unsure of how to relate to him – it was clear that he was no longer a part of their world. Some would sit and stare, putting the burden of conversation on Bill. Others would keep things totally superficial, going on about TV shows, sports, the latest office gossip. The frivolity of this against the backdrop of IVs, monitors, johnny coats and bedpans only increased Bill's feelings of alienation and anger. The world he was once a part of began to seem like a foreign place that he knew was impossible to re-enter. No way back, and no way forward.

8. Signpost: Traversing the Dark Hole

Time and time again, as I walk with people along the Path of Suffering, they describe an accumulation and convergence of emotions (from Signposts 1-7) as drawing them into a deep bottomless pit of desolation and despair. In fact, this is so common that, despite the uniqueness of each person's circumstances, they all describe their experience the same way, equating it with being "sucked into a dark hole."

St. Therese of Lisieux described this "dark hole" in the diary she kept during the final stages of tuberculosis. Her physical suffering was intolerable, and despite her great faith, she too descended into darkness. She wrote: "What would become of me if God did not give me courage? A person does not know what this is unless he experiences it. No, it has to be experienced!" And, to the sisters in her convent she confided, "Pray for those who are sick and dying, little sisters. If you only knew what goes on! How little it takes to lose control of oneself! I would not have believed this before."

So many people I deal with reiterate St. Therese's feelings. Linda, a parishioner of mine, hung between life and death due to serious complications of blood clots in her legs and lungs after a double mastectomy. She shared with me that, "While in the ICU, during the night hours, I was awake so very often and alone, I recall the isolation and desolation in the darkened room with the only noise being the hum of some equipment. I couldn't move. I couldn't turn. It was as if I was paralyzed. And in my aloneness I felt emptiness and vulnerability. I also felt that I was standing at the precipice of an abyss."

Likewise, Bob, another member of our St. James community, expressed his dark hole experience in a personal memoir he published before his death. *Continuing Journey – A Catastrophic Event Doesn't End*

It chronicled Bob's knee replacement surgery in which a mistake was made that paralyzed him from the chest down.

> Bob wrote: "I was in a state of distress that surpassed anything I had undergone until then. I was having increased trouble breathing to the point of having to fight for each breath. It is very much like when I had pneumonia, except I do not have pneumonia. In the past, I would be turning to God for help. I would be asking for strength, for a feeling of peace. God would be very present in my mind. Not so now. I was filled with an unbelievable feeling of despair, a darkness that defied the presence of any light. I tell Terri, my wife, " I don't want to do this anymore." Then I just quit. The thought I held in my mind was not a prayer. I was making a statement to Christ: 'Jesus, kill me, Get it over with. Kill me now.' I was sucked completely into the black hole that had invaded my soul. There is no escape."

The intensity of the dark hole is usually proportionate to your physical, emotional, and/or spiritual suffering. Ultimately Therese, Linda, and Bob emerged from this dark place with a greater sense of peace, faith, and freedom – evidence that the way you walk the path determines how you'll emerge – or not. Despite the emotional and physical exhaustion, loneliness and grief, they prove that there *is* a way to approach even the most desolate parts of the path in a way that is transformative and life-giving.

9. SIGNPOST: ADAPTING TO A NEW NORMAL

Finally you realize that you've reached the point of no return. In the case of a serious or terminal illness, there are even greater losses ahead – from the activities you enjoyed, the food you loved, to your mobility, day-to-day functioning, even what you see as your dignity. You may feel there is no longer anything you can bring to the table. So many simple things you'd once taken for granted – the satisfaction of having completed a full day's work, getting up after a good night's sleep, enjoying a meal, the sun on your face, the sound of the ocean, birdsong in the morning, crickets on a summer evening – how you wish you could make others understand the preciousness they're often blind to. The grief you feel in regard to these impending losses is intense. Practically, you might need help dressing or bathing yourself, might be confined to a bed or wheelchair. You may have to give up living independently, build a routine around treatments. You're continually having to alter your view of what is normal. It's an unpleasant process of constant readjustment that always involves loss – and this is difficult because we all have a natural resistance to change. None of us wants to move out of our comfort zones.

After Richard was diagnosed with ALS he experienced the consistent diminishment of every aspect of his life. Each week seemed to bring another loss – his ability to dress himself, to hold a fork or spoon, to walk unaided. With each loss came a redefinition of who he was, forcing Richard to continually readjust to a "new normal."

10. SIGNPOST: WHO AM I BECOMING?

In light of all this, you must grapple with the sobering question, *who am I becoming?* It isn't about the practicalities or outer trappings of life. This question penetrates the very core of who you are. You may experience the same sense of ambivalence you knew as an adolescent, feeling out of sorts in your own skin. As Jesus said, you can't put new wine into old wineskins. If you do, the wineskins will burst under the pressure.

So, you begin to ask big questions - Who am I, anyway? What is my worth? What was the meaning and purpose of my life? Did my accomplishments really make a difference? Is this honed down version of me my true self? Has everything I've clung to been a façade?

The answers to all the big questions are rooted in the obvious: "What behaviors and attitudes are being manifested as you walk this path? Are you self-absorbed and fearful? Or are you able to walk in freedom and grace? Are you struggling to control the uncontrollable? Or can you surrender it all to a power greater than yourself? Who do you trust – yourself – or God?

YOU HAVE A DECISION TO MAKE

During any period of prolonged suffering you're like a grape being crushed – you'll produce some kind of wine – bitter or sweet. The instinctive reaction is to continue to hang on to what's familiar, to cling to the shell of your former self. Your suffering will increase as you begin to see the futility of your task. This will produce a lot of bitterness – and the old wineskins will eventually burst.

The alternative is to choose a new way of walking (putting new wine in new wineskins). The literal reality of what you're dealing with won't change – but you'll be freer to love, you'll have fewer attachments, and therefore become a conduit for God's love. As you let go and ease into your new reality you'll continue to grieve, but along with grief will shine the first light of inner healing. Your image of God will soften and expand. The outer trappings and concerns of life will become less important, and you'll begin to recognize that the only thing that really matters is love. You'll gradually be able to see life and death as a continuum, as a cosmic and spiritual "yin and yang," each part mysteriously completing the other. Wouldn't we be better able to walk the Path of Suffering with the freedom that comes from wholeness and oneness? With a greater ability to love unconditionally along the journey that leads from life to death?

This is the way of transformation. After tasting this new wine, "dying and rising" will no longer be some abstract theological notion. You'll see that it is actually a life-giving, faith-filled "rehearsal" for your actual physical death. You won't be afraid. And in fact, you'll prepare others for the change that's coming, dispelling their fear along with your own.

The question you'll need to consider is this: Will these natural human experiences along the Path of Suffering cripple you? Or transform you? In the next chapter we'll look at the tipping point between our natural instinctive reactions along the Path of Suffering and the more intentional, yet counter-intuitive loving responses that can radically change the experience for you and everyone you encounter on this ultimate journey.

CHAPTER 3

The Tipping Point

AT SOME POINT in time we all will have to walk the Path of Suffering described in the last chapter – and, in the course of a lifetime, likely more than once. We might find ourselves the patient, or in the role of loved one or caregiver. The question is, what options do we have that can change the nature of this inevitable journey?

Unfortunately, when faced with the crossroads of suffering, standing at the precipice of the dark hole, most 21st century Americans tend to choose the avenue of control that leads to self-absorption. Our instinctive response is to desperately struggle to get an uncontrollable situation under control. We spend every ounce of energy focused on our own misery, obsessed with the situation, and we begin to give days away like candy. More importantly, when we're so radically focused on ourselves we simply won't be free to love. Some of us will persist along this exhausting route until the day we cross the bridge to death.

The other road points the way of surrender, freedom, and love. Choosing the way of love requires a conscious, counter-intuitive decision that might, at first, feel something like giving up. This is one reason why we avoid it. It can also, initially, become a point of contention between loved ones. As they share the Path of Suffering one may be ready to walk the alternate way, the other not. The good news is that regardless of where you are on the Path of Suffering, there's always an access road, an opportunity to cross over to the way of love and surrender. All it takes to alter the route is an openness to the prompting of God.

Keep in mind that walking the Path of Suffering in the way of freedom, rather than control, doesn't preclude being proactive in pursuing the best course of treatment that can provide the highest quality of life during whatever time you have left. On the contrary, it's important to do your due diligence, to explore your options. But when this effort is the *only* focus, when it eclipses everything else – relationships, concern for others, your spiritual life, your opportunities to make meaning of the life you've led, or to do the all-important work of saying goodbye, then you're wagering all you have on a single bet that is guaranteed not to pay you back in spades. Better to keep all things in perspective, and devote equal time and energy to the *way* you decide to walk the path.

DISPOSITIONS ALONG THE PATH

It's important to consider the dispositions you're embracing along this path. These are described on the fulcrum chart, next page. In addition, the fulcrum exposes an often invisible dimension of the path – the fact that there is a parallel unconscious struggle going on between what we call the ego self versus the spirit self. On the left side of the fulcrum you'll see all the attitudes typical along the road of the ego self, or of egocentric control. On the right, those of surrender, freedom, and unconditional love. These are the characteristics of the spirit self.

Notice the behaviors and attitudes indicative of the ego and the spirit selves. If our focus is heavy on the ego, it will be light on the spirit. If our focus is heavy on the spirit self, it will be light on the ego. Keep in mind, this is not an "either or" dynamic. The fulcrum of the self is always in flux, but can be influenced through awareness and intention. Who will you become during your sickness and dying? The choice is yours.

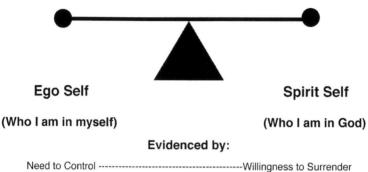

Ego Self

(Who I am in myself)

Spirit Self

(Who I am in God)

Evidenced by:

Need to Control --Willingness to Surrender

Trust in Self--Trust in God

Instinctive, protective reactions-------------------------Intentional loving responses

Holding on---Handing over to God

Unforgiveness---Unconditional Forgiveness

Many attachments--Sense of detachment

Sympathy---Empathy and compassion

Focusing on self-interest--------------------------------Focusing on the interests of others

Feeling separate from all that is-------------------------Feeling one with all that is

Loneliness--Solitude and solidarity

Conditional optimism--------------------------------------Unconditional Hope

Trying to manipulate God----------------------------------Seeing God as loving and merciful

Trying to unravel mystery---------------------------------Embracing mystery

Resistance to change--------------------------------------Openness to change

Denial, resignation, acceptance------------------------Transformation

Dependence on my strength----------------------------Dependence on God's strength

Fear and anxiety--Inner stillness and peace

Self-absorption--Freedom from self

With this in mind, go back and consider the Path of Suffering in the last chapter. Read it twice – once imagining the experience when dominated by the Ego Self. Now envision the same journey through the alternate way of the Spirit Self. Notice how the attitudes and behaviors change. The first is dominated by control and fear, the latter by surrender and love. When in a controlling stance we tend to *react*; when in a loving posture, we can better *respond*.

So, where do you find yourself?

Let's project this a step farther...think of the dynamic between patient and caregiver and/or family members. With these attitudes in mind, imagine the ways this journey can be altered, depending on how each person involved endeavors to walk.

What if both are ego-centric? Can you imagine what the interaction at each Signpost along this path would be like? Although they may care deeply for each other, because the ego dominates, they each struggle for control, causing every imaginable conflict.

Caregiver ⟷ **Patient**
Ego Self   *Ego Self*

Or, if one person is ego-focused, and the other spirit-focused?

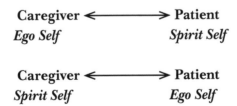

Caregiver ⟷ **Patient**
Ego Self   *Spirit Self*

Caregiver ⟷ **Patient**
Spirit Self   *Ego Self*

This scenario offers a more hopeful shared journey, but when the ego flares, it will be challenging. For the Spirit Self partner, the support of a church community or soul friend is a real necessity to prevent them from tipping the scales back toward the ego self.

But, when *both* parties understand and embrace the power, hope, and, most importantly, the love that the Spirit Self produces, the Path of Suffering can be transformed for everyone involved.

Caregiver ⟵⟶ Patient
Spirit Self   *Spirit Self*

Remember, one's stance is never "either-or." We're much more examples of "both-and," tipping the scales somewhere between the two extremes, the balance always shifting. Often, because of the unpredictability of a disease, we experience loss and suffering in a sort of an ebb and a flow. For awhile we're tipping the scales toward unconditional love, then we hit a setback or other complication. The weight will likely tilt toward control again – our natural instinctive reaction. But by intentionally practicing the art of surrender, we can shift the focus toward love and once again lighten our load.

THE EGO SELF (THE FALSE-SELF) AND THE SPIRIT SELF – HOW THEY TIP THE SCALES

Every living thing is imbued with varying degrees of consciousness. We don't think of a plant as being conscious, yet there is a cellular awareness that draws its leaves and blossoms toward the sun, its roots to water. Human beings possess a more sophisticated kind of consciousness – we're capable of a greater awareness of ourselves and of the ways in which we interact with others and the world. We have many more motivations and desires than a plant or an amoeba. Beyond the basic necessities of life we seek security, affirmation, recognition, the admiration of others, perhaps prestige. We consciously compete with others to excel and succeed. We're brought up with values intended to help us achieve these goals, most of which are necessary in order to make it in our society. As we grow we acquire these *ego strengths* – and this is a positive thing. We need ego strengths to survive in the world, and spend the first forty or so years of our lives striving to develop them. It's important to cultivate the skills, capabilities, and confidence necessary to earn our way, form relationships, and cope with difficulties. It's also normal to seek pleasure, to strive to be successful in our endeavors, and to pursue our interests.

Over time we begin to define ourselves through these ego strengths and accomplishments. We establish our sense of self largely through these outward signs of success – or of failure. We might pride ourselves on being mothers, doctors, crafts-persons, musicians, or classify ourselves as possessing certain distinctive traits – we're creative, or "no-nonsense," financially astute, athletic, attractive or any number of other labels, both positive and negative, all tied to our egos. We use these self-definitions to set ourselves apart from others. *"See, I am uniquely me..."* is what the ego is telling us. The ego will also defend and protect these defining self-images, and will go to great lengths to do so. Keep in mind that anything that is a perceived threat to our survival, self-definition, or self-interest is a threat to the ego self.

This **Ego Self,** although just one aspect of who we really are, can begin to dictate our lives. When we're overly concerned with the ego, when we become attached to our labels and consumed with defending them, we begin to live out of what spiritual teachers refer to as *the false self.* What is false about the false self? It overlooks and often denies the totality of what it means to be human, ignoring our spiritual selves, neglecting the soul. It is the false self that clings to and amplifies hurts, harbors resentment and un-forgiveness, puts us in a defensive posture, and identifies us as victims. If our sense of self-esteem and well-being is built largely on the false self, we easily become self-absorbed. As an illness begins to rob us of our abilities and well-defined roles, we're cast into a panic of self-preservation. The false self desperately strives to sustain life as it is, to protect the personal façades we've worked a lifetime to create. This dynamic can interfere with our ability to learn and grow from our suffering, and prevents us from transforming it into something life-giving. Each signpost along the Path of Suffering strips something from us, requiring us to adapt to a "new normal." If we're dominated by the false self, all our energy will be focused on clinging to the past, to maintain the status quo at all cost. The energy and attention that it takes leaves nothing for anyone or anything else, and actually robs us of the very life we're trying to save.

OUR TRUE SELVES IN THE SPIRIT

The worst part of clinging to our false selves is that we forget that there's another part of us - in fact, the most sacred and beloved part - and that is *who we are in God*. Before we were brought up by our parents, molded by our schools, and pressured by our culture, our souls existed. This true, unalterable self usually gets buried under all the rest. Another way of saying it is that the true self represents who we are when all the trappings of our strivings, insecurities, and overblown egos get stripped away. This true core self is also referred to as the soul or *the Spirit Self*, which is infused with an abiding and unalterable sense of dignity and goodness. The spirit self does not seek praise, distinction, or any other external measure of worth. Unlike the false self, the Spirit Self has no compulsion to compare, compete, to judge, or to win. It is not threatened by others' success, and is unafraid of failure or change. The true self can readily accept the vulnerabilities of life, and encourages a grateful heart in all situations. Nothing can affect the true self in its ability to love because it is one with and in God. This is beautifully expressed in Psalm 139:13:

Darkness is not dark for you,
And night shines as the day.
Darkness and light are but one.
You formed my inmost being;
you knit me in my mother's womb.
I praise you, because I am wonderfully made;
wonderful are your works!
My very self you know.

Because of the tension between the false and true selves, there will always be a battle - the need to control versus the longing to surrender to unconditional love. We're always leaning one way or the other. We

36

struggle between the desire to maintain our separate, unique Ego Selves that we've spent a lifetime building, while at the same time, consciously or unconsciously, yearning to touch into the spirit within, to be a part of all that is. Ideally, to experience what it means to be truly human requires a union or loving dialogue between the ego self and the spirit self. Our spiritual lives and practices should help us to integrate the ego and the spirit into a life-giving balance. (Chapters 16-17 will explore ways to approach this.)

At times, especially right after the onset of great loss - whether a serious diagnosis, the rupturing of a relationship, a tragedy of some kind - the fulcrum will naturally be heavily tipped toward the side of control. It's unavoidable, as we instinctively try to protect ourselves. But we don't need to stay there.

The fact is, like it or not, walking the Path of Suffering changes us even when we don't want to change. The difference is, when the fulcrum is light on control and heavy on love, the changes you'll experience are positive ones. Your vision of life, attitudes, and thinking are different than they were before, tempered by suffering.

Larry, who we met earlier, who'd lost his two daughters in a car crash, experienced this. I worked with him as he traveled the Path of Suffering. In dealing with his loss he struggled with the idea of "putting new wine into old wine skins." True, he had become more compassionate and empathetic – he now knew, firsthand, what it was like to suffer unimaginable loss. But, he persisted in trying to maintain as much of his former "ego self" as possible. He didn't want to let go of his vision of life or of self. It was bad enough to lose his daughters – he didn't want to surrender his identity as well, or let this beat him. He persisted in doing the same old things the same old way, despite the fact that they seemed to be steeped in emptiness and futility. There was something inherently inauthentic in this stance that complicated all of his relationships, particularly his marriage. His wife had changed radically, accepting that she'd never be the same again - she put "new wine in new wineskins." Dealing with Larry's insistence on remaining who he was before became a challenge.

Then, Larry was cast on the Path of Suffering a second time. Diagnosed with a rare lung infection, he found himself hospitalized for three months, teetering between life and death. During that time, he finally let go of the man he used to be. His understanding of the challenges of life had changed still again, and he knew, at the core of his being, that he couldn't go back to business as usual. He'd have to adjust his priorities, attitudes, and thinking, so that his life bore witness to all of the qualities listed on the right side of the fulcrum – the evidence of unconditional love in action. He was stripped down to his essential self, and wanted to learn how to embrace it, to redefine himself as who he was in God. He finally understood what Jesus meant in John 12:24 when he said, *"I say to you, unless a grain of wheat falls to the ground and dies, it remains just a grain of wheat; but if it dies, it produces much fruit."* Clinging to his former self ensured that he would never move forward in freedom and respond to the world with unconditional love. "Fr. Tom," he finally said to me, "I need your help. How do I create new wineskins? I can't do it on my own."

This illustrates the fact that suffering knocks us out of our comfort zones, and forces us to ask, "Do I need something greater than myself to get through this?" We begin to realize, for the first time, that our ego selves were always intended to take a back seat to the true self, the spirit self that can be defined as "who I am in God alone."

By raising our awareness we can, with God's help, throw the weight, in a more consistent way, toward surrendering to unconditional love. Will we fall short? Of course. Even on the way of love we'll all experience what St. Paul expressed so poignantly: *What I do, I do not understand. For I do not do what I want, but I do what I hate.* -- Romans 7:15. The fact that Paul gets outside of himself enough to notice his shortfall is evidence that he can get back, once again, on the way of love.

And so can we. We can choose, again and again, to surrender toward the disposition of the spirit self. As I tell parishioners, "When you fall off the horse, get yourself back on again...and again...and again." Doing so changes the way we walk this path.

At the beginning of the chapter we talked about a fork in the road on the Path of Suffering. Most of us wander along the road of fear and control until we're sick and tired of it. Until we feel as though we just can't go on. When that happens we alter our approach to the path – but first we need to understand how our culture holds us back – and how this makes it much more difficult for us to suffer and die.

When the Ego Self Dominates

When we rely primarily on control, the ego self becomes exaggerated and the spirit self is diminished. Heavy on self, light on God. (See below.)

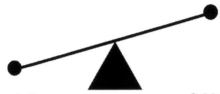

Ego Self

(Who I am in myself)

Spirit Self

(Who I am in God)

Evidenced by:

Need to Control --Willingness to Surrender

Trust in Self---Trust in God

Instinctive, protective reactions-----------------------Intentional loving responses

Holding on--Handing over to God

Unforgiveness---Unconditional Forgiveness

Many attachments---------------------------------------Sense of detachment

Sympathy---Empathy and compassion

Defending self-interest---------------------------------Promoting interests of others

Feeling separate from all that is---------------------- Feeling one with all that is

Loneliness--Solitude and solidarity

Conditional optimism-----------------------------------Hope

Trying to manipulate God-------------------------------Seeing God as merciful, loving

Struggling to unravel mystery--------------------------Embracing mystery

Resistance to change-----------------------------------Openness to change

Denial, resignation, acceptance-----------------------Transformation

Dependence on my strength----------------------------Dependence on God's strength

Fear and anxiety--Inner stillness and peace

Self-absorption---Freedom from self

Conditional love--Unconditional Love

Clinging to your False Self-----------------------------Accepting your True Self

CHAPTER 4

How our Culture Makes the Journey Difficult

MY SISTER MEGGIE'S friend, Rachel, was fifty-eight years old when it became clear that the breast cancer she'd been fighting was gaining the upper hand. She'd already undergone a mastectomy, radiation, chemo and hormone therapy, and been ravaged by a wide range of drugs. Her cancer had metastasized, spreading to her lungs and bones. The aggressive treatment was beginning to feel worse than the symptoms. Her life, once focused on her husband, young adult sons, friends, and work, had now taken a back seat to the disease.

Meggie called and asked if I could meet with Rachel. "She's exhausted, Tommy," Meggie explained. "Ready to give up. She needs you."

So, we agreed to meet. Rachel was home alone, the house quiet. But the presence and vitality of her family was palpable – the baby pictures, golf trophies, the ski gear propped by the back door. Rachel herself, pale, thin, shadows circling her bright eyes, seemed like a ghost of the vibrant woman in the photographs.

We sat down and Rachel sighed. "I've fought the good fight," she said. "Done everything I was supposed to do, one hundred and fifty percent." She stared out the window. "But nothing's worked."

"What's your body telling you? " I asked gently.

"I'm dying," she replied, eyes welling. "I know it. The doctors know it." She glanced at the beautifully framed family photo of her, her husband and sons. "But they keep telling me I need to fight. Not give in. That I can beat it."

"But, what do you think? "

Rachel leaned back in the chair and closed her eyes for a long moment. Then she looked at me. Her gaze was penetrating. She took a deep breath. "It feels as though I'm missing something. That there's a dimension of this that's beyond my grasp. I sense it, I want to take hold of it – because if I do, I know I'll finally be able to *do* this."

"Do what, Rachel? "

"To *die,*"she said. "I'll finally be able to die. But Bill and the boys just won't let me."

Rachel had tapped into what's at the heart of the dying process – despite her family's refusal to go there, she'd been drawn toward *mystery.* Slowly, surely, her awareness of something greater than herself and her situation had summoned her. For a while, she'd stood in the tension between wanting to go back to what life had been, and moving on to the next phase. Yet her family, who naturally wanted to keep her alive, refused to acknowledge any other option than to continue the fight. Rachel began to feel increasingly alone. Her family, friends, community, medical establishment, though well-intentioned, simply were not willing to stand with Rachel in the greater mystery of her dying.

All the "big stuff of life" – creation, love, birth, suffering, death – are steeped in mystery. Mystery can call forth awe, wonder, and light – a sense of the miraculous. It's what makes us gasp, step back, and marvel at the chance meeting of someone you later fall in love with, or at the birth of a child, a totally unique creation, or the dawning of a new day.

But there's another side of mystery – we also gasp, step back and wonder when faced with the darkness of suffering and loss. Without a doubt, the experience of sickness and dying involves dealing with the most challenging mystery of all, evidenced by people continually asking me, "Why this is happening, Father? How did it come to this? What will happen next? "

All unanswerable questions.

In my many years of working with families standing in these situations, one thing has become increasingly clear: our culture does little to help us deal with the mystery of death. In fact, cultural values actually make it much harder to die than it need be, as it inflates the ego self. When faced with *any* great loss, we Westerners have a particularly difficult time emotionally, mentally, and spiritually. To better understand, let's reflect on the role and function of culture in our lives.

By their very nature, modern societies strive to analyze and control mystery. We look to science, logic, data, and empirical evidence to explain what we can't get our heads around. This isn't a bad thing. Obviously, tremendous progress has come from advances in science and technology. These innovations help bring prosperity, a sense of security and order.

Still, despite modern innovations, true mystery cannot ever be adequately grasped, explained, or controlled – it can only be entered into. And so, the problem begins.

HOW OUR CULTURE DICTATES OUR ATTITUDES TOWARD LIFE AND DEATH

Besides sharing customs, values, and beliefs, all cultures influence its members to deal with living and dying in ways intended to sustain the common good. Culture's main function is to protect against forces that might threaten its existence, and to encourage members to thrive by protecting a reasonable amount of self-interest. We see this clearly in our own Declaration of Independence, defining our inalienable rights to "Life, Liberty, and the Pursuit of Happiness."

AMERICAN CULTURAL VALUES

Our country's institutions, through a consistent and repetitive socialization process, shape our upbringing, and create the lens through which we view the world. In subtle and not-so-subtle ways, they strive to maintain themselves by molding the masses, by promoting and facilitating the productivity of its citizens. We're rewarded when we align ourselves with their vision, and marginalized when we don't. The more we fit in, the more we experience a sense belonging, and are afforded the rights and opportunities of the culture.

We get a strong sense of cultural ideals through symbols, rituals, and celebrations that are systematized through our institutions – governmental, educational, economic, recreational, and religious. One powerful example is sports – the "Golden Calf" of our society. I'm always amazed how the Superbowl has become an unofficial national holiday that showcases our American values of nationalism, militarism, and capitalism – beginning with the National Anthem as a call to battle, complete with military jets soaring overhead, the immense American flag stretched across the field. And then there are the clever Superbowl commercials. Between the four million dollar price tag for a 30-second slot, and the two million dollar production costs, a one-minute ad can cost a whopping ten million dollars. All of this is held up, celebrated, and observed by over 111.5 million people! I can't think of another event with that kind of impact. It serves as both a mirror and a reinforcer of what we hold important.

The Superbowl is just one powerful symbol that represents 21st century American values. We strive for success. Achievement. Competition. Self-reliance. Productivity. We applaud the "self-made" woman or man, the accomplished individual who overcomes any and all obstacles. We respect people who are always in control. We fight to win, sometimes at all costs. We need to be #1, to amass as much wealth and as many possessions as we can, to dominate in all things – our military budget is powerful proof of this. (According to the Peter G. Peterson Foundation, the U.S. currently spends more on defense than the next ten highest countries *combined*.) We are a nation of winners.

Amassed wealth, as evidenced by houses, cars, vacations, and diverse portfolios equates with success and security. We're fascinated with the lives of the rich and famous – just walk through the check-out line in any supermarket and see the collection of magazines and newspapers that scrutinize the lives of Hollywood celebrities, sports stars, royalty, and political figures. Consciously or unconsciously, we look up to them, because they represent what we hope our children can strive for and become. After all, isn't this the American dream? We often dedicate our lives to the pursuit of it. This striving can result in chronic, obsessive busyness that prevents us from embracing higher levels of consciousness cultivated through solitude, silence, simplification of lifestyle, and the sense of surrender necessary for transformation.

> *Do not conform yourself to this age but be transformed by the renewal of your mind, that you may discern what is the will of God, what is good and pleasing and perfect.* – Romans 12:2

What I've seen, over and over, is that while we include God in our lives in varying degrees, it's often as a nicety, or as a sort of insurance policy. In fact, we depend less on God, and much more on our own ability to deal with life. We're taught to suck it up, persevere, to use our willpower and personal resources to overcome our difficulties.

The media continually fuels our need to attain, and then hold tightly to these things we believe we need in order to be happy. We develop strong emotional dependencies on all we've acquired. The thought of losing any of our possessions is deeply disturbing. The objects of our desires are called *attachments*. We become attached to our wealth, possessions, lifestyles, and relationships. The late Jesuit priest, Anthony de Mello, in his book: *The Way to Love* has said, "The tragedy of an attachment is that if its object is not attained it causes unhappiness. But if it is attained, it does not cause happiness – it merely causes a flash of pleasure followed by weariness, and it is always accompanied, of course, by the anxiety that you may lose the object of your attachment."

A friend of a friend, who was suffering from a terminal illness, provided a sad and powerful illustration. His wife called me, distraught. Her husband was failing fast, growing weaker by the day. While she was at work, he'd somehow rallied the strength to get himself out of the house, and returned home with a new car, and not one, but two expensive Italian leather jackets. After the initial rush of power and pleasure, the man plunged into deep despair. These small trophies were intended to provide a sense of validation, and to contradict the reality of his imminent death. What they brought was emptiness. An extreme example, but it clearly shows how the movement of sickness, dying, and death exacerbates our desire for and anxiety around inordinate attachments.

Our Culture's Fascination with Death

At the same time, our culture seems to be fascinated with death in a voyeuristic way. Turn on the TV at any hour, day or night, and you'll find programs dramatizing every imaginable kind of death. Police dramas about murder, medical examiners performing forensics, gang violence, mafia wars – the list is endless.

Others take it beyond entertainment to lived experience, engaging in extreme sports, dare-devil feats, or continually striving to live on the edge. We're intrigued with anyone looking the tiger in the eye, because the culture tells us, if we're strong enough, bold enough, brave enough, smart enough, and have enough resources, we can stare the tiger down, grab it by the tail, and control it. Unconsciously, the message here is that death can be beat. But, sometimes, to our surprise, the tiger bites...

Implications for Sickness, Dying, Death

Mystery? Sickness? Dying? Death? These fly in the face of our societal values. We simply cannot tolerate what we can't control. Subconsciously, death is the ultimate failure.

It makes sense then that the way in which we respond to any great loss is largely due to our conditioning. Our reactions are expected and predictable. To respond in any other way would fly in the face of the ideals we've been brought up to embrace.

In light of all this, when we find ourselves or a loved one suffering with a chronic or terminal illness, what are we to do? How are we to cope? We're encouraged to rally all our resources, search out and line up any and all allies for the fight ahead.

Of course, our first line of defense will include the tools we've used successfully in the past - our natural coping mechanisms.

What are they, and how do they work?

CHAPTER 5

Three Ways of Coping with Sickness and Dying: Denial, Resignation, and Acceptance

EVERY LIVING THING comes equipped with a thrust for life and a natural drive toward survival. Fight or flight, face-off or retreat. When a threatening encounter is unavoidable, a porcupine raises its quills, a skunk lifts its tail, a cornered dog attacks. This is the most primal of all instincts, one not unique to the animal kingdom.

Even as highly evolved human beings, we share this natural response with all God's creatures – but there's a difference. You and I bring other dimensions into play – our superior intellect, our emotions and ego, our capacity for spirituality. These empower us to function in a more sophisticated way, but also add layer upon layer of complexity to the basic fight-or-flight instinct. In addition, there's an innate human impulse, an expansive energy that propels us not only to preserve and lengthen life, but to deepen the experience of living. If we're open to it, this generative movement leads us from the surface of life and draws us to a higher level of consciousness. This inclination can lead us beyond the most basic responses to life's losses – from *denial* to *resignation*, to *acceptance*, and most importantly to *transformation*.

This movement demands an ongoing and ever deepening process of surrendering to our losses, our vulnerability, and, ultimately, our own mortality. Due to myriad fears, anxieties, and cultural pressures, we often resist this God-given thrust that seeks to move us forward, and we can easily get stuck in one stage.

In this chapter we'll look at the first three phases – denial, resignation, and acceptance - and the cluster of inherent defense mechanisms we depend on during this time. We turn to these "first responders" whenever we feel vulnerable. Denial, resignation, and acceptance shield us from suffering, enabling us to be physically present, but psychologically detached, protecting the ego from any threats to our survival, security, sense of belonging, self-interest, and self-esteem. These defense mechanisms serve as buffers against perceived danger, protecting us from hurt, stress, pain, or loss, and are essentially positive - the default settings of the human psyche that kick in as needed. These natural defense mechanisms keep us afloat by focusing on *control.*

In the course of our normal day-to-day living our natural defense mechanisms, when used sparingly, serve a valuable purpose, giving us some breathing room in which to collect ourselves in order to respond to challenges in a healthy way. However, when faced with bigger problems, when our health or life is threatened, we tend to double and triple down on these natural responses. Instead of using them as transitional tools, we start relying on them, minute-to-minute, just to get through the day. In essence, we retreat to our "internal control center," building a wall of defense around ourselves. While this wall attempts to shield us from anxiety, it also isolates us, deadening our ability to enter deeply into relationships, numbing our awareness, distorting reality, and hindering our ability to experience the simple joys of living. The tremendous amount of energy it takes to maintain this level of control leaves little for anything expansive or life-giving. We substitute one kind of suffering for another. The fact that our "go-to" strategies cease to deflect our suffering only increases our compulsion to try to control the uncontrollable. We continue to experience mental anguish, emotional distress, spiritual desolation, and physical pain, creating a spiral of suffering that only intensifies. The energy and concentration required to maintain this wall forces us into a stance of radical self-absorption that cuts us off from everyone and everything that brings meaning to our lives. It hampers open, honest, and loving conversation and prevents us from being free to give or receive love.

HOW DEFENSE MECHANISMS PLAY OUT DURING SICKNESS AND DYING

Throughout the journey of sickness and dying it's normal to rely on the tools that have helped us in the past. Understanding the nature of defense mechanisms and acknowledging the need for these natural coping tools can allow us to be a little gentler with ourselves or empathetic toward those we love who might be relying on them as they strive to come to terms with a new and frightening reality.

What follows are some examples of how the common defense mechanisms often manifest themselves during sickness and dying. There are many defense mechanisms – we'll focus on the ones I see the most. Recognizing these behaviors in ourselves and others can elevate our awareness, and provide a ray of hope that there can be, eventually, another, healthier way to respond.

Denial

This first coping mechanism dominates the entire initial phase of the journey. When in denial we refuse to acknowledge a traumatic situation. As we face something we perceive as catastrophic to the world as we know it, we can become like the proverbial ostrich with its head in the sand. At a certain level, we recognize what's happening, but refuse to acknowledge it or to consider the implications. This helps us avoid dealing with the powerful emotions inherent in the situation. Before moving to resignation, acceptance, and transformation, we typically spend a good deal of energy denying the reality before us. This stage allows us some psychological space where we can begin to adjust to a 'new normal'. Denial can last for hours, days, months, years, or, in the extreme, until the moment of death.

A young family man named Mark was dying of cancer. I got a call from his wife, Jennie. She was feeling frustrated and alone. In addition to her grief over her husband's illness, she felt shut out of his internal world. Mark would obsessively involve himself with the lawn, working on his car, maintaining his daily routines. He'd talk about sports or politics – anything but the difficulty he was dealing with. The emotional intimacy they once shared was gone. There was a huge elephant in the room that Mark skirted around at all cost. As long as he maintained some semblance of his day-to-day life he could pretend that he wasn't dying. And the effort and stamina this took left him exhausted.

Mark was in denial. He became so totally self-absorbed that his wife, his children, his parents and siblings all became invisible to him. For them, it was as though he was dead before he died. Even as he entered into hospice care, Mark refused to acknowledge his impending death. He passed away without ever saying goodbye to his wife and his sons. Jennie's grief was not only about the loss of her husband, but about feeling shut out of his world when he needed her most.

ANESTHETIZING OURSELVES

Sometimes, when facing a traumatic situation, we feel an overwhelming need to blunt or cap the emotions that threaten to tear down the protective walls we've erected. In striving to sustain a state of denial, we seek numbness through a variety of addictive behaviors. Increased alcohol use, abusing prescription medications, using illegal drugs - all amount to self-medicating. A nightly glass of wine becomes an entire bottle, the occasional use of pain-killers escalates into a round-the-clock necessity – not to address physical discomfort, but to hold powerful emotions at bay. Excessive shopping, exercise, eating, cleaning – any of these can be used to anesthetize ourselves against whatever it is we're trying to deny. We seek the blind oblivion that allows us an escape from the reality we most want to avoid.

Resignation

In time, the consequences of our illness (or other serious situation) become more and more intrusive. We're eventually forced to alter our daily routines, and adjust many aspects of our lives. Perhaps we have to stop working. We might require help with our personal caretaking, or the maintenance of our home. For most of us, moving from denial to resignation is rooted in the realization that "I just can't do this anymore." The paradox is this – we're in denial because more than anything else, we want to *live*, but the very effort to keep reality at bay, to sustain the illusion that we're not going to die, creates its own life-strangling kind of hell. There's a sense of stagnation and a pall of despair that becomes more oppressive than the reality of the disease. The capped emotions eventually push to the surface. This "uncapping" is a function of our natural thirst for a higher level of consciousness and freedom, and the resulting flood of awareness gradually ushers us from denial toward a state of *resignation*.

When we resign ourselves to this new reality we finally acknowledge the facts and understand the prognosis. We might hunker down and resist, or gather all our resources and begin to fight in earnest. Some strive to find a solution, overcome the obstacles, battle against fate in any number of ways. For others, resignation is accompanied by varying degrees of negativity, anger, and/or depression. It also activates a variety of alternate defense mechanisms that allow us to perceive the reality, but mask the suffering.

INTELLECTUALIZING

As I sat next to Judy at her 60th birthday party she leaned over to me. "Fr. Tom," she said, "I just hit the lotto." Her tone of voice didn't match her message. I turned toward her, eyebrows raised. She looked away and went on. "I just got diagnosed – inflammatory breast cancer – the worst kind." Shook her head. "But I'm determined to defy the odds."

The information supplied by her doctor and the results of her online research confirmed it – most patients don't survive beyond five years, even with aggressive treatment. In the months that followed, Judy focused intently on her treatment, tests, medication, holistic and alternative therapies - at the exclusion of everything and everyone else. She felt driven to "figure it out," talking about it incessantly. 'Why" and "how come" became her mantra. Perhaps it was the stress of her job all these years...or maybe she'd been exposed to a chemical of some kind? Was it her diet – the extra thirty pounds she carried after the children were born? Birth control pills? Antiperspirants? There had to be a logical *reason*. A clue that would lead to a solution, a cure.

There is certainly nothing wrong with a patient taking an active and informed role in his or her treatment. In fact, it's important to do that. But, there comes a point when the diagnosis has been made and the prognosis is clear. When that prognosis is terminal, it's critically important for a shift in focus to take place. I always say, "It's as important to prepare to die as it is to fight for life. But you can't really do both at the same time."

– No one can serve two masters. He will either hate one and love the other, or be devoted to one and despise the other. --Matthew 6:24

Intellectualization is a means of holding the deeper emotions at bay, to avoid consciously addressing impending loss and the difficulty of bringing closure to the relationships that matter.

Judy's health rapidly declined. I visited her many times. "Judy," I'd say. "It's time to begin the work of dying." She would either pointedly ignore me or angrily reply, "I told you - I'm going to beat this!"

She died finally, a year and half after her diagnosis. During that time she was never able to get in touch with her deep feelings or to share them with her family. In that way she died alone, with her loved ones surrounding her bed.

It begs the question – *Does it have to be this way?*

EMOTIONAL DISSOCIATION
Everyone was amazed at how well Kate took her cancer in stride. Upbeat, positive, and seemingly open about her situation, she was an inspiration to all. "Honestly, I'm doing just great," she'd say. "I'm exercising

regularly, doing wheat grass, kale, and blueberry smoothies to build myself up. I believe in the power of positive thinking. I know the prognosis, but I'm going to extend my good days for as long as I can – live each day to the fullest."

At first glance, Kate seemed the ideal patient. She manifested what we all view as the most positive and mature response. The problem was that she'd completely cut herself off from the range of emotions naturally associated with the challenges of treatment and the threat of death. As Kate's health deteriorated her husband became more and more frustrated with his wife's resolute assertions that she was doing fine. While she admitted that she had a terminal illness, she refused to allow herself to experience the losses she was dealing with. Sure, she was going to die, but not right now. He wanted to talk about what their life together had meant, discuss one daughters' college graduation, another's wedding which would likely be taking place without her. But, it was never the right time for that. Kate could not go there, refused to say her goodbyes or make amends, to take stock of the life she'd lived, and to prepare her family for her impending death. She would not allow herself to face her losses, vulnerability, and mortality and the emotions that run through these end-of-life experiences. Doing so would open the emotional floodgates, rendering her helpless.

Does it have to be this way?

ANTICIPATION

Cathy, suffering from a serious congenital heart problem, would look at her husband and teenaged daughters, her siblings, friends and co-workers, and anguish over the fact that their lives would continue on without her. Thoughts of everything she'd miss – milestones, birthdays, weddings, grandchildren, growing old together with her husband – the overwhelming sense of sadness threw her into a depression that debilitated her and everyone around her.

Michelle, dealing with M.S., spent her days worrying, projecting far into the future. She imagined what her suffering might be like, her loss of mobility and independence. She imagined herself in a wheelchair, unable to care for herself or her children.

While anticipation can be used in positive ways – for example, putting into place practical strategies now that might be helpful later – Michelle and Cathy indulged and immersed themselves in incessant negative thoughts and projections, responding to them emotionally as though they were happening in the present moment - to the point that they robbed themselves of the days, months, and years of relative health and happiness that could have been better spent with loved ones. So, in addition to dealing with illness, Michelle's and Cathy's obsessive thinking threw each of them into a state of crippling anxiety.

Does it have to be this way?

DISPLACEMENT

Jack and Louisa had been happily married for 35 years when he was diagnosed with Parkinson's disease. The illness took hold and Jack degenerated quickly, experiencing tremors in his hands, stiffness in his muscles, and an overwhelming sluggishness in his movements. The couple, golf enthusiasts, had bought a condo on the golf course, and had spent many carefree days golfing with friends and neighbors. But now swinging the club was becoming impossible and Jack would sit in the cart watching the others. One day, after a golf tournament, Louisa came to see me and told me the following story. While at dinner as Jack was lifting his coffee cup his hand shook violently, causing the coffee to spill over the white tablecloth. A while later, dessert was served, everybody congratulated Louisa on a birdie she'd shot on a particularly difficult hole. Jack uncharacteristically made a cutting, disparaging remark about his wife that was met with an awkward silence around the table. It seemed as though, along with the disease, Jack had developed a mean streak. "Father Tom," Louisa said, tears welling in her eyes. "Jack's become a different person. I try to help him, but everything I do is wrong. He's critical. Cruel even. Not the man I married."

As often happens, the caregiver had become the silent victim of the disease. Jack, frightened and frustrated, felt like a pressure cooker of powerful emotions, and displaced his anger on a safe target – his wife.

This too begs the question – *Does it have to be this way?*

Acceptance

Often, people fight their way through denial, become resigned to the reality before them, and gradually move toward the more peaceful state of *acceptance*. (Although some get stuck in resignation and stay there until their deaths.) Those who have moved to acceptance decide to make the best use of their time, prioritize their relationships, and keep anxiety and sadness at a minimum. They accept the fact that they have a terminal illness and work to keep things as normal as possible. Enjoy what they can. Debra, the mother of three children, suffering from leukemia, lived out the days she had left in a state of acceptance. She was generally upbeat, did her best to shield her family from the realities of her illness, and was intentional about where and how she spent her time. Her first priority was her immediate family and several friends that she allowed into her world. Family and friends were continually impressed by what they saw as her strength and positive attitude – her daily Facebook posts of her smiling through her treatments, her focus on living every moment to the fullest. On most days Debra felt a sense of peace in coming to terms with death. She would leave this world her way, setting the rules for her dying, and move through her bucket list to the best of her ability. She'd try to express whatever she needed to those she cared about, and put in place a support system for her husband and children. She used her time to best advantage, "tying up loose ends," and taking stock of the life she'd lived.

But, from time to time, when the news was not positive, Debra would slip back into fear, regret, and worry – the by-products of *control*. These she kept largely to herself.

While acceptance is certainly preferable to resignation, it is still often rooted in the ego self. Still a way to, on some level, try to control mystery.

NOW WHAT?

We've seen how the values of our culture force us into a posture in which we feel compelled to maintain control at all cost, and therefore to desperately depend on our defense mechanisms. We lose any sense of harmony between our bodies, minds, and souls. The dis-balance that occurs when any one of these crucial aspects of our humanity become either exaggerated or dismissed results in great stress and anxiety. It also intensifies physical pain and emotional and mental anguish. Instead of restoring balance through awareness and acceptance, we continue to struggle to maintain control and manipulate reality. Like the Dutch boy who wouldn't remove his finger from the dike, we're terrified that if we step back, even a little, the waves of disaster will come crashing over us and we'll perish.

At some point, we begin to realize that perhaps this is just too much to try and handle on our own. The next logical step is to turn to others for care and support. At the end of the day, don't people say, "blood is always thicker than water? " More often than not, whether we really want to or not, we look to family.

CHAPTER 6

——————— ⟨———⟩ ———————

Let the Games Begin

WHEN DAVID WAS dealing with terminal cancer, I was called in to see him. As soon as I arrived it became clear that his adult daughter Ellen had designated herself as the family "gatekeeper." When I began to talk honestly with David, Ellen stepped in, bringing the conversation to a hasty close, insisting that I was to simply "give him a little blessing." David looked at me, sighed, and shrugged. In speaking with David's son, I learned that Ellen closely monitored not only all visitors, but the information that came in and out of the house in regard to their father's disease. She also became the go-between in relation to her father and his doctor, controlling how much information her father "could handle." Ellen strictly maintained this triangle, keeping the rest of the family at arm's length. As I always say, "When the situation is being dealt with from a stance of control, especially in the context of family systems – then, let the games begin." This dynamic, in which information and individuals have limited access to the family, is called a closed family system.

FAMILY SYSTEMS

Like David, anyone dealing with a serious, chronic, or terminal illness naturally turns to family for support. (Signpost 3 on the Path of Suffering) With the clear focus on the patient, it's easy to forget that he or she is part of a larger family system. Every person within the system not only affects the others, but is affected by them, both positively and negatively. Any disruption in the system has an impact on *all* of the members.

With the focus on the family member who's sick, it's easy to overlook the fact that the primary caregivers within the family are on the Path of Suffering along with the patient. Dealing with a loved one's illness kicks up fears and anxieties in regard to their own vulnerability, losses and mortality. How the patient and the caregivers individually deal with the illness significantly impacts the entire family. The way they relate to one another can make the journey on the Path of Suffering much more difficult - or much more life giving. Will this illness become an ongoing crisis, or an opportunity for understanding, compassion, and transformation? Naturally, we'd all say that dealing with an illness in a life-giving way is what we would want for everyone involved. But, often this can be a challenge.

Engrained family patterns of relational dynamics are established over generations, and therefore difficult to alter. The way we interact as a family is determined by our experiences growing up, our ethnic background, religious beliefs, and the culture we live in. While all of these influences are powerful, perhaps none is as powerful as our individual family values and rules. Family interaction, introduced and reinforced throughout our childhoods, becomes the internal program that dictates the way we relate to others. And whenever the family system is threatened with a chronic, serious, or terminal illness, we have a tendency to revert to these almost innate attitudes and patterns of behavior.

It's important to take an objective look at the way your family functions. How do its members interact? Is there open, honest, and loving communication within the family? What are the influences – both spoken and unspoken - the messages, values, perceptions, attitudes, and prejudices that formed family members over the years? What are the predictable responses during times of emotional turbulence? When things go wrong, is the immediate family forthcoming with extended family, friends, and neighbors? How resistant is the family to change?

FAMILY BOUNDARIES – OPEN OR CLOSED?

The first dynamic that all family members (and anyone wishing to help these families) need to be sensitive to is the issue of boundaries. Boundaries determine the level of openness the family can tolerate within its operating system. Additionally, these boundaries control who is allowed to enter into the family system, and to what extent. They also determine the degree to which family members feel free to relate to the outside world and regulate what information is allowed in and outside the family unit. As family members and outside caregivers try to relate, they need to gain a sense of how permeable the family boundaries will be.

When the boundaries are permeable the information flows more liberally in and out of the family system. Family members and others can move and communicate more freely and without reservation. This is a characteristic of an open family system.

Dee and Denis were active parishioners at St. James for many years. They were great stewards of God's gifts, serving the community in a multitude of ways. Denis retired, the couple traveled extensively, and finally decided to move closer to their children. They sold their house in town and bought another home in upper New York State. Denis and Dee were so excited and happy to start this new journey together. As they were settling into their new home, I received the following email from Denis, which he allowed me to share here:

Hi Fr. Tom,

This morning, our lives turned on a dime. The results of a biopsy on Dee's liver came back positive for carcinoma. Over the next couple of weeks, we are likely to have a lot more tests to determine what, if anything, can be done. Could we ask you two favors? First, keep Dee in your prayers. Secondly, could you send us the draft of your book? It looks like we are going to need it.

-- Denis

I called Dee and Denis and we spoke for a while. They were anxious for our St. James community to hear the news and to offer whatever support they could. A day or so later the following email, with a very wide distribution list, appeared in my inbox:

Dear Family and Friends,

Here is the update we promised after our first visit to the oncologist this morning:

Dee has stage 4 cancer of the liver, meaning that it is metastasized and not operable or curable. The prognosis is that if she elects not to do chemo, she will live less than six months. If she takes chemo, it will add months, not years, to her life. If she tolerates it well, there is an outside chance that she has 24 months left.

Whether the cancer started in her liver or migrated there from somewhere else is unknown at this point. On Friday, she will have a PET scan to determine if tumors are found elsewhere in her system. The most likely candidates now are lymphs and esophagus. Next Thursday, she will have an endoscopy for her esophagus. At that point, we will know the best course of action for the chemo, and we will start it shortly thereafter. If she tolerates it well, she will continue. If not, quality of life trumps longer life, and she will stop the treatment.

We will also be seeking a second opinion.

At this point, she is suffering discomfort in her stomach - which is reasonably tolerable. Her energy/stamina is not bad: she has good days and not so good. Nothing she eats seems to agree with her. But we take our walk every night, and we hold each other and cry a lot. And try to keep our wits about us.

Thank you for all the prayers and all the love. We ask you to continue to keep her in your prayers. Sorry, we are adding some of you to the mailing list for the first time, and this is the first you've heard about this. Please spread the news to those you think would want to know.

-Denie

Clearly, they were operating within an open system. There are many benefits associated with this, particularly the outpouring of loving support from friends near and far, as evidenced by the next group email:

Hello all,

Dee has been completely overwhelmed by your responses to the recent emails on her health situation. So have I. Thank you for all your love, and all your prayers, and for all the memories you have shared with us.

And thanks to those of you who have forwarded the previous emails to others. Unfortunately, our e-mail list is limited, and we don't know who you forwarded the e-mails to. So we ask you to do it again...forward this one to the same people.

So here is the situation: nothing substantial has changed. Dee has undergone about eight tests, and we have traveled to Sloan Kettering in NYC (number 2 rated cancer hospital out of 901 in the USA) for a second opinion. The tests have tended to confirm the diagnosis we told you about in the first emails. She had "innumerable tumors" in her liver, and the source of the cancer seems to be her bile ducts. The "second opinion" oncologist confirmed that she is in Stage IV, meaning that the cancer has spread to multiple sites throughout her body. It is not operable or curable. This doctor's prognosis was just a tad better than the first: with chemo, the median survival period is about a year. That means we have a 50-50 chance of her living longer than a year.

So, Dee will be starting aggressive chemo treatments on Sept 29th, and we will see how they affect her. We don't want to trade off quality of life for a slightly longer life - so we may or may not continue them after Christmas, depending on how she responds. That is also the time we will have another CT scan to see if the chemo has had any affect on the tumors. Both oncologists were pretty blunt: there is a 30 to 40% chance that the chemo will shrink the tumors, but a zero chance for a cure.

In the two and a half weeks since the last e-mail, we have learned a lot about what she can eat without making the discomfort worse. Unfortunately, it is limited to yogurt, Boost shakes, Kashi cereals, and occasionally some cooked fruit and power bars. Anything that requires bile for her digestive system to process has a negative effect - so all meats and anything with oil or lots of carbohydrates in it is out. The good news is that she has stopped losing weight, and now weighs what she did in the sixth grade. We are still learning, consulting, and exploring what kinds of things she can eat, and there is a possibility that the chemo may in fact increase the number of things that she can tolerate.

She is in good spirits most of the time. And she still has more good days than bad. As I am writing this, she is cleaning the bathroom. She's not about to let me take these things away from her until it is absolutely necessary.

On our way down to Sloan Kettering, we were playing the sound track to *A Chorus Line,* and the song *What I Did for Love* brought us both to tears. "Kiss today goodbye, and point me toward tomorrow." It's a song about not having regrets for how you lived your life. And we both realize how blessed we are to not have any regrets. That, more than anything, brings a special poignancy to our most frequent prayer, which continues to be "Thank you God for right now." And we are getting much better than we ever were at enjoying our 'right nows.' Even the tears.

Please continue to keep us in your prayers. And thank you all again for your overwhelming love - and for standing with us "in the center of something rare and fine."

-Denie

It's interesting to note that the third signpost along the Path of Suffering is "Dealing with Family and Friends." You see in the above emails how Denis and Dee are striving to do that. Their boundaries are very open. Denis also shares his thoughts and feelings quite freely. His expressions of appreciation for the prayers and support of so many that has sustained them is heartfelt and genuine.

Another benefit of connecting to others in an open way is that the gifts received go both ways. Everyone who opened their email was moved, touched by their honest vulnerability. It stirred not only empathy, but compassion. Recipients were inspired by Denis and Dee's faith, by their devotion to one another, and were challenged to reevaluate their own lives and to "live in the now" more consistently.

Other families' boundaries are less permeable, and therefore the flow of information in and out of the family is more constricted. To outsiders, these families often appear self-sufficient and private, closing ranks very quickly when some crisis arises. This is more typical of a closed family system. There are very legitimate reasons why families may, at times, restrict the boundaries of their system – for example, parents often tighten the limits around children or teenagers in order to protect them or keep them safe. Another example of this was when Liz was in the final stages of breast cancer. Becoming fatigued by well-meaning visitors, she decided she needed to close the boundaries a bit in order to spend what little quality time she had with her immediate family. Her family was sensitive to this need and closely monitored visitors.

Keep in mind that most families are not simply "this way or that way." They fall somewhere on the spectrum between open and closed boundaries. In both examples – Dee and Denis (open) and of Liz (closed) what allowed each family to function in the most life-giving way was open, honest, and loving conversation. These kinds of conversations are what I call the "lubrication" that keeps families flexible, responsive, and sensitive to all of their members.

When both open and closed family systems are navigated through *control* (or dominated by the ego self) these conversations are impossible. If a member or members are ego-focused it's impossible to communicate openly with others. A common example of this is in the home of an alcoholic. In Barbara's family dynamic, it was clearly understood that she was not to discuss her father's alcoholism and addiction to prescription drugs with anyone. The tacit agreement was that this was something that should be dealt with privately. This cloak of silence was exhausting to maintain. Each family member suffered "alone together" which caused an even greater sense of isolation and emotional suffering. There was resistance to outside intervention, making it nearly impossible for the family to get any kind of professional help or counseling. Even as he died from the effects of this condition, no one spoke about the elephant in the room. Barbara and her mother were so successful at guarding this family secret that decades after her father's death, when Barbara broached the subject with family and childhood friends, they were all shocked to learn the truth of those years.

Another taboo subject for many closed family systems is death. The terminal illness is only discussed obliquely, any conversation focusing on treatment and the practicalities of care. Inquiries from others outside the family unit are met with vague responses at best, and at worst, families may avoid others at all cost in order to eliminate the possibility of probing questions. This is essentially a reflexive protective mechanism, the automatic ingrained response of those in closed family systems in an effort to side-step the anxiety surrounding the situation. What begins as a protective instinct ends up causing even more stress. Besides the stress of dealing with the illness, members of tightly controlled closed systems have to process and deal with the pressures of avoidance and denial.

This kind of control inhibits and restricts the kinds of loving conversations that preserve the best interests of all of its members.

EMOTIONAL BONDING - CLOSE OR SEPARATE?

All relationships within family systems can be categorized somewhere between being emotionally close or emotionally separate. How much do family members bond with one another, and how much individual autonomy do they maintain? Bonding within families occurs when there's a history of consistent care for one another that allows each member to feel as though they belong, that the family is a safe place to be. This kind of nurturance creates an atmosphere in which open, honest, and loving conversations can occur. Consistent care, along with loving conversations, results in an environment in which mutual trust and emotional intimacy flourish. At the same time, healthy families encourage each member to thrive in their own unique way, so that they can develop a sense of self apart from the others. When nurtured within the family system, members can remain bonded while maintaining their own sense of autonomy – in other words, creating an atmosphere of both unity and individuality. It's natural for there to be tension as the needle moves between bonding and autonomy. Family members need to constantly adjust and adapt in order to remain emotionally close without becoming either *enmeshed* or *disengaged.*

Sometimes, individuals become so dependent on other family members that they become "enmeshed" – unable to think independently or make decisions without input and approval from the others. For example, two sisters might pride themselves on being extremely "close" and "connected," but in reality are unable to think about or deal with difficulties independently. They must talk constantly, hashing and rehashing every aspect of every situation, leaving no room to breathe or reflect. They literally talk a subject to death, and are paralyzed without the input of the other. This dynamic creates an illusion of intimacy, when, actually, the relationship is rooted in an exaggerated sense of dependence. All sense of individuality is lost. Each member sees him or herself as primarily a "Smith" or a "Jones" - the collective identity always taking precedence. Individuals in enmeshed families are usually perceived by outsiders in this same way. If a family member tries to exert autonomy they can be scapegoated and marginalized by the other members – becoming the "black sheep" of the family.

The opposite of enmeshment is disengagement. When the situation gets too hot to handle, one or more members may emotionally "check out." Each sees her or himself as essentially separate from the rest. There is little sense of family bonding or of familial connectedness. This disengagement might be active or passive-aggressive, but, either way, the disengaged person will not give of him or herself emotionally. "I just can't deal with it," becomes the mantra for disengagement. The disengaged family member holds his or her self-interest above all else, and takes a reactive, protective stance in regard to the family. This results in cut-offs and estrangement.

Whether enmeshed or disengaged, these extremes can create huge tensions when the family has to face the challenges of dealing with a serious or terminal illness. Both ends of this interpersonal spectrum are rooted in *control*. This type of control eliminates the possibility for open, honest, and loving conversations that enable families to work together and navigate the challenges of a chronic, serious, or terminal illness.

FAMILY ADAPTABILITY - FLEXIBLE OR STRUCTURED?

Family systems can also be structured or flexible. What routines are in place which ensure that day-to-day life can move along smoothly while accommodating the needs of the patient? Too much structure (rigidity) puts stress on everyone involved, as diseases are unpredictable and require extra attention as needed. Also, a terminal illness disregards routines, schedules, and responsibilities, and must be dealt with as situations arise. A flexible system allows for give and take, for schedules that can be adapted to the needs of both the patient and caregiver.

But, in the extreme, flexibility can degenerate into chaos. In chaotic households no one's needs are being met, there is no sense of order or predictability. This too can cause great frustration and confusion.

I visited Rick, perhaps a week away from death. His sick room was wide open to family, friends, and neighbors. They congregated around his bed, chattering amongst themselves, making small talk. People came and went. The "out of control" atmosphere of constant chaos prevented any kind of intimate, honest, loving conversations. Later Rick said to me, "Fr. Tom, I can only say this to you. I just wanted to tell them all to get the #*!* out of here! It was painful!" Refusing to draw healthy boundaries can become another kind of control, committing to chaos as a shield against being real with one another.

OTHER FAMILY DYNAMICS

There are still other dynamics that can affect the family system. I often find that individuals within the family structure regularly over or under-function. How often have you seen a situation in which one family member seems to do all the work? These over-functioners may feel as though no one else can do it right, while at the same time feeling resentment toward the rest. Others in the family may under-function, often because they feel that no matter what they do it's just never good enough. These under-functioners also experience resentment at the system that won't allow them in. Rather than discussing these roles, and the feelings associated with them, both over and under-functioners begin to feel like victims, and the vicious cycle continues.

Another dynamic is *triangularization* – when one family member will not communicate with another, and uses a third member as a sounding board. This forms an unhealthy triangle, in which one member becomes the outsider. Sometimes one point of the triangle can be the disease itself. Rather than speak about what they're feeling or about the state of their relationship, two family members instead focus all of their interaction around the disease – the symptoms, and the treatment.

The same thing can occur between the triangle of the medical team, the family, and the patient – the doctor communicates to the family, the family screens and distorts the information, and then delivers their carefully controlled message to the patient. These triangles are formed when open, honest, and loving conversations are not taking place, and in which members are trying to closely *control* the situation.

WHAT TO DO?

In order to proceed in a way that's healthy for the family, there's a need for what I call **relational lubrication**, to help families decide whether and how to adjust their boundaries. Would more openness help? Might some limits on engagement outside the home be useful? This allows families to modify their boundaries and patterns of relating in response to whatever a particular situation calls for.

The "oil" that lubricates the system, that allows for flexibility without chaos, and connection without enmeshment is *open, honest, and loving conversation.* And what undermines this communication more than anything else is when individual members tip the fulcrum toward the ego self. When approaching these challenges primarily from a stance of control, when the ego self dominates, then let the games begin.

Eventually, most families in this situation come to realize that somehow the culture has failed them, their defense mechanisms have come up short, and their families haven't been able to mobilize in ways that hold back the onslaught of suffering.

So, now what?

At this point, like a soldier in a foxhole, out of ammunition, many of us decide to turn to God.

CHAPTER 7

The Shattering of Naïve and Reasonable Faith

As we're forced to stare into the face of death, God may suddenly become a much higher priority. We may cry out for help, desperately looking for some power greater than ourselves that can somehow, some way save us. This may be the first time we've actually paused to consider who this God is, practically speaking, and the particular image and experience we have of God will dramatically affect the way we reach out in faith. Those with a mature faith seasoned by suffering will eventually move through resignation toward a state of acceptance – and if they tap deeply into this faith it can be transformative. However, this level of mature faith is something few of us have intentionally nurtured. In the "green times" when involved in the busyness of life, most of us feel little need for any kind of consistent, intentional spiritual pursuit. But when we receive death's calling card, we often take stock and call our faith into question.

As we look at the first two fundamental levels of faith to help determine where we find ourselves, keep this in mind: None of us is as spiritually mature as we'd like to be. So, approach this discernment with a sense of gentle realism. The point isn't to chastise ourselves over the state of our faith lives. Rather, like using a map, we want to be able to pinpoint a starting place (YOU ARE HERE) so we can begin to move toward our destination of recognizing our oneness with God. Remember – even the disciples of Jesus, who spent years with him, who heard his teaching firsthand, proved ill-equipped to grasp and live his message until after they experienced his death and resurrection. Being real about where we stand is the gateway toward deepening our faith – a process that will empower us not only to live well, but when called, to die well.

THE FIRST TWO LEVELS OF FAITH

When life turns on a dime there are two fundamental levels of faith we may try to tap into – both rooted in the ego self. Our faith, along with our natural coping mechanisms, becomes a "team of first responders." Adding God to our defense team makes us feel more confident in our ability to get things under control. The problem is that when the ego self is dominating it keeps us locked into these first two levels of faith, making mature spiritual growth a challenge.

Throughout most of our lives many of us stand in the doorway of faith, so to speak, afraid to pass through. We stand at the portal, uncomfortable, preferring the empirical world to spiritual mystery.

A few brave souls venture across the threshold, but most of us are afraid. We believe God is *out there somewhere,* but from the refuge of the doorway, God seems distant and remote. This makes it easy for us to project an image of our own making onto the face of God - one that's workable for us. It might be God as a power to be feared, or, a "nice" God who can be reasoned with. Either way, we feel that if we do and say the right things, we can get God to do what we want - to control the difficult situation we find ourselves in. This God we've created is mostly all about what *we* want to see happen, and is only embraced so long as things go our way. In reality, there's more of *us* than anything else in this God of our own making.

NAÏVE FAITH

I remember a mother whose son, in his forties, was dying. She attended mass daily and considered herself a religious person. She'd spent the last year fervently praying the rosary, saying novenas, offering mass intentions for her son's recovery. When I went to the hospital to visit the young man just before he died, I found her in a nearby conference room, out of control, furious about her son's impending death. She raised her hands, looked to the ceiling and cried out, "God! Why are you doing this to my son? "

She had faith, but it was on a very basic level. It was a *naïve faith*. She used her religious practice as a barter system – if I can appease God in some way, God will do what I want. Prayers and devotions in exchange for control. Religion as an insurance policy against loss of any kind. She felt she could control God, and therefore control life, through her well-intentioned practice. At a certain level, she believed that if she said her prayers, went to mass, and tried to be good, that nothing bad would happen. In fact, she might be able to generate a miracle, based on the fervency of her practice and devotion. She didn't understand that the "fear" of God mentioned in the Old Testament actually translates as awe and wonder - to be fascinated and captivated by the wondrous mystery of the living God. Instead, the God of her making was a demanding judgmental figure. If you mess up, this God will punish you.

To take her credo a step further, under this God's rules, his subjects will go to heaven if they're good, or to hell if they're bad. With naïve faith there's a tendency to take normal guilt and intensify it into a punishing, neurotic guilt. This can lead us toward becoming religiously scrupulous, multiplying prayers and devotions, in order to accumulate enough "points" to get us into heaven. There's a tendency to think dualistically, to become self-righteous, to see things as right or wrong, black or white. This religious and moral certainty usually leads to severely judging ourselves and others.

Possessing naïve faith brings us a false sense of security. The difficulty with this level of belief is that it crumbles when we're faced with more difficult and complex situations. When difficult situations happen, it's a call for us to go deeper into the mystery of God. If we choose not to, we become spiritually stuck. We feel guilty when life takes a difficult turn, because, clearly, it must be our fault – if only we'd prayed and gone to church more often, read the Bible, if only...if only... This type of guilt causes us great anxiety when we, or someone we love, is in the dying process. Practicing naïve faith becomes exhausting, so it's no surprise that often people give up, or just fulfill what they see as their basic obligation – the equivalent of completing a checklist for admission into heaven. Where everything will be nice. Perfect. Happy.

But, is that naïve, utopian ideal enough to transport us or a loved one through the many transitions of suffering and surrendering that mark the dying process? Are any of us really eager to say goodbye to those we love, or exchange the world we know for a distant unknown heaven, however joyful and peaceful – even in the presence of God?

REASONABLE FAITH

I consistently run into people who say that the reason they don't worship or pray is that they "get nothing out of it." When we have *reasonable faith* we feel that any spiritual practice needs to make us feel good. In the past we might have engaged in religious practices in order to produce a sense of satisfaction, peace of mind, fulfillment. We go to church because it's meaningful and affirming, and we feel good when we leave (as long as it isn't too long!) Our worship services need to be entertaining – the homily has to be good, the music has to move us. Outside of church we meditate and practice yoga because it quiets us and affords us a feeling of overall wellbeing.

None of this is "bad." In fact, on the contrary, why shouldn't our religious practice and/or church-going provide these benefits? (Perhaps if more care was given to the quality of the service churches offer, more people would fill the pews - but that's another issue altogether!)

The God of reasonable faith is not to be feared – this is a *reasonable* God. It is a God in whom we can place great expectations. But when things aren't going well, this God disappoints.

Ed, a young family man dying of prostate cancer, resigned to the realities of his disease, tormented himself with unanswerable questions. "Why me? I know guys who cheat on their wives, fathers who don't pay child support. I'm a good husband and father. I work hard. It's not fair!"

He was angry with God, with life, and spent all of his energy trying to figure out why this was happening to him. This was his constant refrain – God was just not being reasonable.

The reasonable God is also a deity-on-call. Always benevolent, always meeting our needs. When we reach out, he'd better be there for us, to provide what we believe we need to be content. We "co-opt" and use this God to justify our pursuits that we believe will make us happy. This dynamic exists individually and as a society. As a whole, our culture sees God as the deity of our prosperity. Instinctively we know that our relationship with God can't be a one-way street, therefore we want to please Him – but, on our terms. We do this by being "nice" and striving to do what we "should" do, as long as it doesn't cost us much. We refuse to look at the complexity of issues, such as social justice, or war, because the ramifications of that might affect our bottom-line or rock some of our basic beliefs in exaggerated ideals such as patriotism, capitalism, freedom.

So, without too much introspection, we embrace a reasonable God who will justify our values and pursuits. As long as God meets our expectations, we like and follow him, if God doesn't, we're disappointed, and will gradually put him on a back burner.

FLIP SIDES OF THE SAME COIN

Whether we have a naïve or a reasonable faith, it's important to recognize that they're just two sides of the same coin. When life turns on a dime, we find ourselves constantly flipping the coin, hoping one side or the other will magically work for us. We do believe, but at a very primitive, fundamental level. This faith might be sufficient when life is going our way, but will begin to shatter when we have to deal with the serious brokenness of ourselves and the challenges life presents.

So, what happens if we discover that our faith has proven insufficient in the face of great loss? Or in the midst of sickness, dying, and death? Typically, we regress, doubling or tripling down on our efforts to cope and control. We experience spiritual darkness – a sense that God is distant or absent. When this happens we might give up any practice of faith. Or, if we continue to practice, we scale it back to a minimal level. (Just in case, we're covered, we maintain our membership in the club, preserving our ability to become active as needed.) Experiencing a serious difficulty, we may have a tendency to blame and get angry at this God. He is not playing by our rules.

When denial and/or resignation weds itself to naïve and reasonable faith, it creates an illusion of control that's difficult to break through. We fall into greater self-absorption, the sense that life is slipping from our hands increases, and we confine ourselves to an obsessive pattern of worry, control, worry. This cycle creates a whirlpool effect, spiraling us into a dark hole – so much so that the very life we seek to save begins to feel like a prison.

At a time when we know we have a limited number of days at our disposal, it's important to look at this self-imposed prison – however painful that might be - so that we might find a way to break free, live out the rest of our days in freedom, mature faith, and love.

CHAPTER 8

The Prison of Self

*"A human being is a part of the whole that we call the universe,
a part limited in time and space. We experience ourselves, our
thoughts and feelings, as something separated from the rest—a
kind of optical illusion of this consciousness. This illusion
is a prison for us, restricting us to our personal desires and
to affection for only the few people nearest us. Our task must
be to free ourselves from this prison by widening our circle of
compassion to embrace all living beings and all of nature."*

– ALBERT EINSTEIN

ALL OF US, because of our brokenness and vulnerability, have experienced what I call the **"Prison of Self."** It's sometimes so common we become blind to it. And, if we can't recognize that we're in the Prison of Self, then we're not going to be able to do the work required of us during sickness and dying that is most life-giving, not only for ourselves, but for those standing vigil with us. It's hard enough being wrapped in the bandages of loss or illness, without being "self-wrapped" in this prison. This self-absorption will cause greater emotional distress than whatever physical pain we may encounter. Just as Jesus called Lazarus (John 11:44) from the grave saying, *"Untie him and let him go free,"* he's calling to us. If we don't recognize the prison we're in, we can't possibly break free to live fully the days we have remaining.

PROCEED GENTLY

I ask you to be patient as I take you into the Prison of Self. It's important to see the totality of what "incarceration" is like. As you move through it, some of the images may touch into your story. Aspects may resonate with your own experience, and, when it does, you may feel a little depressed, overwhelmed, even fearful. If you recognize any of these behaviors in yourself, or a loved one, it may be difficult to face, for the first time, the invisible bars that have held you (or them) prisoner. But recognition, experienced through the lens of gentleness and understanding, can become the key to unlocking the prison doors that lead to freedom.

How, you ask, could a person be in prison and not know it? This personal prison is actually so prevalent in our culture that at least some aspects of metaphorical incarceration are, more often than not, the norm. We accept our shackles as part of what it means to live in the world – and just about everyone we know shares them. But once in awhile we see someone who seems somehow freer, lighter, more open and able to love than we are. In light of this, we might feel a hint of anxiety, wondering, as we look at our own lives - is this all there is? Though our vital signs may be strong, these alone do not make a life. Facing a significant loss, chronic illness, or an impending death causes us to take stock. Have we given away days, weeks, months - even years or decades languishing in the Prison of Self? Have we died before we are dead? And if so, is it too late? Too late to experience what it means to live freely and joyfully, to be fully alive? Trust me when I say that living one day in true freedom, regardless of your physical state, is better than simply existing through an extended jail sentence. Don't waste a moment bemoaning what's been lost. Instead, take the first steps toward breaking free.

As we take this journey into the emotional and spiritual jail of our own making, hang in with me, though it might be unsettling, even disturbing. Let me share that anguish with you, and with it, hope - for there *is* a way out of prison. In fact, I've been in prison myself, as all of us have. And the gateway toward liberation is awareness – and selfless love.

WHAT DOES THE PRISON OF SELF LOOK LIKE?

Each area and aspect of the prison represents a feeling, attitude, behavior, or response that occurs when we lock down and focus all our energy trying to *control the uncontrollable*. This effort to control is rooted wholly in the ego self, and the ego-driven behaviors and attitudes intensify. The use of coping strategies (defense mechanisms and primitive faith) increase and are fueled by the fact that we're stuck in a situation that seems hopeless.

PRISON ENVIRONMENT

The environment in the Prison of Self contributes to our inability to see reality for what it is, altering our perception of ourselves and others. The walls are lined with curved, warped mirrors like the ones in a carnival fun house. As prisoners, we're drawn to these mirrors, and as we look into them a voice inside whispers, "Mirror, mirror on the wall, who do I see most of all…"

The answer is, we see only ourselves – but not our true selves. Whenever we look in the mirror, we see a **distorted image** – we call this the **false self**. We mistake our accomplishments and our possessions, the various roles we play in work and family, for our true identity. The distorted mirrors reflect back the superficial window-dressing that we've cultivated and scrupulously groomed – things that, if taken away, would leave us wondering who we really are.

Jamie, a marathon runner and health fanatic, lived a "perfect" lifestyle – exercise, organic foods, and possessed the exceptionally lean, muscled body and golden good looks that come with it. So when he was struck with a debilitating stroke, his image of self was shattered. Who was this person hobbling along behind a walker? Jamie was lost, mistaking his self-designed identity, admirable as it was, for his true inner self.

Occasionally, our reflection in the prison mirrors frightens us. We get a fleeting sense that perhaps there is someone else beneath the surface. These flashes of insight can inspire desperate and compulsive attempts to "find ourselves," yet our distorted images persist. This tiresome search for self eventually wears us down, and we begin to believe that the distorted image of the false self is who we really are, effectively limiting any ability to grow or change.

Ask yourself – how do I define myself? Who am I outside of that definition? What are the things I couldn't bear to lose? Of course we all want to hold on to the things we've accomplished or achieved. But, when faced with any significant loss (of a dream, a relationship, financial security, reputation, loved one, or life itself) we'll be forced to come to terms with a stripped down "self" that has little to do with the accouterment of the life we've made. Recognizing our true selves, our value and identity in love alone, is a process that can only be undertaken *outside* the walls of the Prison of Self.

PRISON WINDOWS

The windows in the Prison of Self are barred and tinted. Looking through them, our view of the world is altered. Instead of seeing the whole picture, all we notice is what people and the world are *doing*, or *not doing* for us. We place great expectations on others. When Loretta's mother was ill, and Loretta would stop to visit after an incredibly hectic day at work, often times the first thing her mother would say was, "It's about time you got here." Her mother never asked about Loretta's day. She only saw her daughter in terms of what she was able to provide, killing any hope of an authentic and meaningful relationship. True, her mother was confined to a nursing home, but it was actually the Prison of Self that cut her off from the joy of living.

THE PRISON CELL

In the metaphorical Prison of Self we retreat to our cells to protect ourselves from further pain caused by others. The cell provides a place to hide, to withdraw from family and friends, to effectively push them away. In this way we feel safe from anyone who might touch into our hurt and cause more pain. There's also a wing of the prison designated for solitary confinement. Here, inmates can stay, isolated from others, for extended periods of time.

Alex, whose wife of fifteen years divorced him, spent the next ten years in the safety of his cell, in solitary confinement. He turned away from the couple's old friends, cutting himself off from any and every reminder of his former life. He became cynical, deflecting any attempts at relationship. His cynicism became the key that kept him locked in his cell of pain and hurt, preventing any possibility of healing and freedom.

THE PRISON LOUD SPEAKER AND TVS

Do we find ourselves stuck inside our own heads, constantly obsessing about some aspect of our lives – perhaps a relationship, an ongoing issue at work – or maybe a chronic or terminal illness? As human beings, equipped with sophisticated brains, a certain amount of objective internal processing is normal. But, in prison, this inner rumination snowballs into radical self-absorption, robbing us of the ability to really see and hear others or to appreciate the world around us.

Imagine the prison loudspeaker, always broadcasting repeated negative messages inside our heads. It runs almost constantly, the announcements reiterating and inflating every worry, over-analyzing every imagined or real transgression against us. Regrets, mistakes, feelings of guilt over the past replay over and over, tormenting us. The loudspeaker also amplifies pointless questions such as 'what if,' 'why not,' 'if only'... It intensifies our fear of loss, resulting in a habitual cycle of anxiety in which we rationalize, bargain with fate or with God, redouble our attempts at will-power and determination, and finally collapse in defeat.

Besides the loudspeaker, there are also TVs that are constantly on, allowing inmates to lose themselves in the programming. What they watch, over and over, are two channels – one broadcasting reruns of scenes from the past, causing viewers to obsessively relive and question past events, hurts, disappointments, decisions, and relationships. The other channel features futuristic fantasy, projecting everything that might happen in the days, weeks, months, years ahead. It's easy to become habitual watchers – and regardless of the channel, the programming prevents viewers from *living in the present.*

Sheila, diagnosed with uterine cancer, was tormented by her internal prison loudspeaker and futuristic TV programming. Statistics for her survival, treatment options, visualizing all the things she'd lose, imagining her future pain and suffering – the litany that constantly marched round and round her head totally dominated her consciousness. She finally recognized the extent to which her inner voices were controlling her while her four-year-old granddaughter was visiting. Sheila sat outside, watching the child play in the sandbox, chattering happily as she moved the sand around. At one point the little girl said, "Right, Grandma? Right? " Sheila realized she hadn't heard a single word her granddaughter had said. She'd been physically present, but emotionally absent.

Haven't we all experienced this – at work, at a party, at a family gathering - going through the motions while the prison loudspeaker blares in our heads? Been distracted or dismissive with others because we simply couldn't see or hear them? We've all inadvertently pushed others away, totally preoccupied with our own internal loudspeaker. As our inner voices scream we become deaf to the voices of others. When this happens you know you're in the Prison of Self.

OUR PRISON GUARDS

Of course there are prison guards to prevent you from escaping. The guards promote the belief that it's safer to exist in prison than it is to risk being free. They are the people in our lives who want us to stay the way we are, even when it's not working any more. The guards in our lives realize that if we change, they might be forced to change as well. They'll keep the status quo at all cost, doing everything in their power to preserve what is, even as they complain about it. They can't imagine how to relate to you in another way. These are the family members who undermine your diet, the friend who discourages you from applying for a new and challenging job, a spouse who refuses to go to couple's counseling. After all, guards would lose their positions if the inmates got out of jail.

THE UNIFORMS WE WEAR

When inmates arrive in prison, they're issued one of six types of uniforms. The thing all of the uniforms share is that they are, in some way, shape, or form, woven of rage.

Anger, in and of itself, isn't a bad thing. There's an energy in all of us that thrusts us toward living life to the fullest. When we become stuck in a situation from which we see no way out, this life force produces anger to help get us "unstuck." It's a positive force intended to propel us toward change. But when we perceive change as frightening, we tend to resist it, gravitating instead toward the same old familiar, if ineffective, strategies that keep us stuck. When this happens, the positive nature of anger changes into a negative force called hot anger or rage, directed at self and/or others. The alternative is that we "cap" our rage, using every ounce of energy to keep it in check. This "caged rage" often results in depression.

Now let's take a look at the variety of uniforms we put on as we enter the Prison of Self, using the lens of gentle realism. As we recognize these uniforms and the negative behaviors that define them, it's important to keep in mind that the wearer is *stuck*, unconsciously transmitting their pain to others.

THE UNIFORM OF RAGE

Some people dress themselves day in and day out entirely in **hot anger** or **rage**. Everyone tiptoes around the person clothed in rage – it doesn't take much to set him off. You know someone you love is wearing the hot angry uniform if you find yourself walking on eggs around him/her, or scrambling to "fix" a situation that will surely set him/her off. Their responses are disproportionate to the situation. The rage-clad person is highly critical and often harshly sarcastic. Sometimes their criticism or sarcasm is passive aggressive – it comes under the guise of humor. Often times caregivers and family members become the target of this rage.

Another variation on this belongs to those who have a compulsion for "telling it like it is," and constantly feel the need to "set people straight." They often inflict hurt on others, hurling a cutting or critical remark because, after all, they asked for it. Chronically angry people usually have a chip on their shoulders. They won't let anyone get away with anything, and find themselves watching for circumstances where someone might take advantage. At the first hint of a transgression, they lash out.

THE DEPRESSIVE UNIFORM

Some prisoners will avoid acknowledging their rage at all cost. They find angry outbursts distasteful and upsetting, and refuse to behave in that way, despite what they may be feeling inside. The alternative is that they slip into depression. All of their energy is used to cap the hot anger within. Since their emotional resources are being used to hold back rage, there's little left for anything else. They have a hard time engaging. Nothing seems to matter.

DRESSED AS A VICTIM

This uniform clothes the inmate as a *victim,* and shouts, "Poor me." The wearer expects things to go terribly wrong, after all, they always have. When dressed as a victim, the person always sees his or her situation as worse than everybody else's. They're always waiting for the other shoe to drop, and seem almost satisfied when it does – at least their preconceived notion about their victim-status has been validated. Victims, by their very nature, seldom ask about others. You see them in the supermarket and head for the next aisle, hoping to avoid their most recent list of complaints.

Barbara's mother was never happy with her life. She resisted change, feeling she was powerless to initiate it. She saw other people as lucky, in fact, prefaced many observations about life with the words, "Other people…"

Once Barbara brought her mother and a friend to San Diego, a place her mother had dreamed of going. They went to the beautiful old Hotel del Coronado and sat on the terrace overlooking the ocean having a cocktail. Her mother looked around and said, bitterly, "Hmmmph. I guess this is how the other half lives…" Barbara looked at her and replied, "Mom – you're here, are you forgetting? " Even in good times, some people just can't step out of the role of victim.

THE ARROGANT UNIFORM

Sometimes people turn their victim uniform inside out. The reverse side of the victim suit is *arrogance*. The person clothed in arrogance doesn't see him or herself like other ordinary people. "After all," he might shout, "Do you have any idea who I am? I deserve better! I don't have to tolerate this!" The Arrogant Uniform fits the person who is demanding, relentless in his/her self-promotion and/or self-glorification. They defend their "rights" at all cost. Their entire being proclaims, "It's all About Me!" They know it all, and you can't disagree or offer another view. In actuality, their arrogance is generally commensurate with a deep-seated sense of inferiority - the inflated sense of self, an extreme compensatory tool.

DRESSED AS A PLEASER

At first glance, this uniform is the most appealing. It's the *pleaser* design. People who don the pleaser uniform work hard – over-functioning - putting themselves out for others, striving for perfection, usually wearing a smile and projecting an agreeable, can-do attitude. They feel as though no one can do things better than they can, and thus discourage others from lending a hand. All of this over-functioning is rooted in the belief that they can get the recipient of their efforts to finally come through and give them whatever it is they need. However, when they don't get the recognition, affirmation, or validation they feel they've earned, they often change uniforms and slip into a subtle sheath of rage or depression.

Marie had spent almost ten years of her life caring for her mother who was in a slow decline toward death. People said Marie was a saint, working round the clock, providing for her mother's every need. However, when family members or friends offered help, Marie declined – after all, she was the only one who could do it right. Marie's mother was sharp-tongued and critical, and despite everything Marie did, her efforts always somehow fell short of what her mother expected. In the end, when the elderly woman finally died, Marie's husband thought it would spell a sense of relief and liberation. Instead, beneath the veneer of a smile, Marie became bitter, resentful, and passive aggressive. Her anger at never earning her mother's approval spilled over into other relationships. She displaced most of this anger onto her husband, jumping on his smallest misstep, real or perceived, her responses always disproportionate to the situation. Her husband could never do anything right, and was baffled by his wife's continual blaming game. She had, in effect, become her mother.

THE MANIC UNIFORM

Lastly, there's the *manic* uniform. This garb can look drastically different, depending on the day – one day the wearer is obsessively involved with an idea, an activity, or a project, running at full throttle, with an abundance of energy and overly focused excitement. Then, dramatically, it all changes and the person becomes emotionally flat, disinterested, tired, depressed.

Harvey was an over-the-top sports enthusiast. He'd gear up for the weekend, plan for his series of games. Before, during, and after he was the ultimate fan, excited, engaged, shouting at the TV, cheering. The outcome of the game meant everything to him – in fact, it was the only time he seemed alive. When the game was over Harvey would slip into himself, withdrawn, depressed, tired – until the next game.

Like Harvey, Caroline also used a basically insignificant activity to make her feel alive. She'd step into her manic uniform and head to the mall, experiencing a high when shopping, unlike anything else in her life. But, almost before she got the bags in the door, her excitement dissipated, and she flat-lined again until her next shopping excursion.

Once inside the prison walls - regardless of the uniform we wear, despite where and how we spend our time, no matter which roles we play - our minds, hearts, and spirits essentially go to sleep. This emotional slumber dulls our senses to the point that many people live and die as inmates. Father Anthony De Mello, author of *"The Way to Love,"* reinforces this understanding:

"You need to realize that you are surrounded by prison walls, that your mind has gone to sleep. It doesn't occur to most people to see this, as they live and die as prison mates. Most people end up being conformists; they adapt to prison life. A few become reformers; they fight for better living conditions in the prison, better lighting, better ventilation. Hardly anyone becomes a rebel, a revolutionary who breaks down the prison walls. You can only be a revolutionary when you see the prison walls in the first place."

IS THERE A WAY OUT OF PRISON?
If you find yourself in the Prison of Self, is there a way out? Admittedly, breaking down prison walls isn't easy. With no hope of transformation, and acknowledging little value in suffering, some may resign themselves to the pain of this emotional and spiritual hell. Others may consider using assisted suicide as a form of escape. It might be rationalized that doing so spares not only the patient, but their families as well. Death is seen as the solution to a problem – a stance that completely dismisses the deeper, more surprising truths about life, family, faith and love that can only be fully realized in relation to and from the perspective of the end point, however painful. We have to walk through it. The decision to

take one's own life can obliterate the lessons and legacy left in its wake. When Bob (whom we met in Chapter 2) said, in regard to the black hole, *"There is no escape."* he was in a place in which his suffering was greater than his faith. But he would learn and testify to the contrary as he persisted along the Path of Suffering. This book proclaims and gives witness to the fact that there *is* a way out of the dark hole and a way out of prison – that fear and despair can give way to greater life, can reveal profound truths and surprising gifts.

Do you find yourself in prison? If so, congratulations. It means you're human – vulnerable and imperfect. Once you recognize this in yourself, you can begin to act with greater compassion and tolerance – to embrace yourself, others, and the world more freely, with the gentle touch of understanding born of pain.

The question is, once we find ourselves in prison, must we resign ourselves to a life sentence? Is there a way to turn off the loudspeaker, trade in the uniform, break out of these prison walls to reclaim the joy of living for whatever time we have left?

"This is the struggle of every person — be free or be a slave." – Pope Francis

Conversion – Moving toward the Spirit Self

"Conversion is a grace: It is a visit from God."

– POPE FRANCIS

CHAPTER 9

Breaking Free from Prison

ONCE WE BECOME aware of our status as Prisoners of Self we can no longer ignore the shackles that impede our ability to live and love. We experience a pervasive sense of unease, and begin to see that the natural coping mechanisms we've relied on have only constricted our lives.

At the same time we have no idea what will replace these former lifelines. We begin to feel a pulsation pushing and pulling us to something greater - that we're inching toward a *conversion* experience.

People sometimes talk about their "conversion experiences" as though they were struck by lightening and – *voila!* Thrown off the horse like St. Paul, picking themselves off the ground, renewed and changed. I suppose this happens for some people, but it isn't the norm. For most of us, conversion isn't neat or quick. It's the pivot point, the launch pad toward transformation, *the awareness that the way we've been approaching life is no longer working.* Conversion leads us into a messy mix of vulnerability, resistance, vacillation, discomfort, retreat…a chipping away of what has been, creating a space for something new. An unraveling of the ego self that begins to tip the fulcrum away from control toward surrender and unconditional love.

Conversion is difficult. It is, at the very least, a three-step process that involves **Dying, Death, and Rebirth.**

Dying -- dismantling or shattering of what is
Death -- the realization that there's no going to back to what has been
Rebirth -- an unknown future that we can't even imagine, that will only gradually be revealed.

Another word for conversion is *metanoia*. It means, literally, to turn around. It begins with the realization that the way we've been living is becoming stagnant and no longer serving us well. To experience metanoia requires us to move from the surface of life, to a higher level of consciousness – an openness to stand in mystery. The paradox is that metanoia can only come as we relinquish control. The process is counter-intuitive, requiring us to let go, when every instinct tells us to hold on even more tightly. It is at the heart of the movement of dying, death, and rebirth.

THE GENERATIVE THRUST OF CONVERSION

In the course of a lifetime there are many situations conducive to "turning around," to seeing things in a new and deeper light. When we're walking the Path of Suffering experienced during any major loss, what drives us from denial to resignation to acceptance is a movement of conversion. Some resist this thrust, pitching a tent and living in a state of perpetual denial, while others begin to let go and become resigned to the reality they face. When this new reality begins to feel too constrictive, another opportunity for conversion presents itself. Will we persist in a posture of resignation or allow ourselves to be propelled from resignation toward acceptance?

Every loss, every "letting go" presents a chance to move deeper into the mystery of life. And ironically, some of the greatest opportunities for conversion occur when we're faced with chronic, serious, or terminal illness. In order to embrace our own sickness and dying with a greater sense of freedom and peace, the necessary first step is to face our *vulnerability, mortality,* and *losses.* These are the three core issues we've been conditioned to avoid.

As I entered middle age I had to face a number of circumstances that began to undermine my basic assumptions about how life worked and where I fit into it. As a result, I became aware of the necessity for ongoing conversion – forcing me from the mindless, fast-paced superficiality of my life toward the slow process of relinquishing the behaviors that had put me into the Prison of Self in the first place.

See if my experiences resonate with your own.

VULNERABILITY

I was 39 years old. For three years I'd been commuting to New York every Friday for graduate studies in counseling. I was also a teacher and a Spiritual Director at a large Catholic high school. On weekends, I was assigned to help out a local parish with masses and confessions. Almost every Sunday I presented wedding preparation classes to engaged couples (Pre Cana) throughout the diocese. In between, I filled my calendar with a lively social life. There was no time for "meals" – I'd eat junk food, on the run. I struggled with some of my relationships. I filled my days with activity in order to avoid reflecting on any of this.

One night, I woke up sweating, my heart racing. An overwhelming sense of panic and impending doom paralyzed me. I was sure I was having a heart attack.

The first thing I did was say an Act of Contrition – just in case. The fear of hell was still part of my life. Somehow, I got up and dressed. Silly as it sounds, I didn't want to die in my pajamas. I sat, read Bible passages. I tried praying with some favorite Psalms. I said to myself, "Whatever's going to happen is going to happen." I never called 911. On some level I must have understood that this was something other than a heart attack – either that, or I had a secret death wish.

A realization slowly dawned on me - I was having an anxiety attack. Me - Superman - who could keep so many balls in the air that Barnum and Bailey had started calling! I had never experienced anything like that before. I wondered if I was losing my mind. It was such an overwhelming, terrifying feeling. I was unable to shake the anxiety, but it did lessen and I managed to somehow get back to sleep.

Early the next morning, I called a good friend who was a psychotherapist and we talked for a while on the phone. That helped a bit. We met later and he referred me to another therapist whom I began to meet with regularly. He helped me realize that the anxiety was a warning sign – the way I was living and processing life wasn't working anymore. He helped me see that I'd been over-using my natural coping mechanisms, anesthetizing myself. It wasn't propofol or valium. My drug of choice was work, frenetic activity, busy-ness, and control. I kept myself in constant motion to avoid experiencing emotions or healing any of life's wounds. These I kept in close check. I was skimming the surface of life. I'd become a workaholic.

My therapist told me I needed to stop - to begin to pay attention and experience, at a deeper level, what my emotions were trying to tell me. He helped me to recognize that even in my priesthood – my vocation - I'd actually embraced my father's shadow self by becoming what he'd wanted to be – a priest. This was the only way to get on my father's agenda, to be important in his eyes. I began to wrestle with many aspects of my life, especially my priesthood. It seemed that everything was coming undone, spiraling out of control.

Over time, my anxiety became less overwhelming, but there was always an edge of nervousness that would flare. I remember some friends threw a party for my fortieth birthday. I came to the party, feeling good, but all of a sudden, the anxiety ambushed me. All I wanted to do was go upstairs and lay down. I knew it was rude, even bizarre, but I didn't care. I could hear the people downstairs having a good time, while I isolated myself. It was painful, but I felt powerless. Toward the end of the evening, they called me down to open my gifts. I went through the motions as quickly as I could and made a hasty escape.

For a number of years, these anxiety attacks would come at different times for no apparent reason. I was functioning, handling all my responsibilities, but I was self-absorbed. The intellectualizing – insight overload and the constant chorus of voices inside saying, " I want to go back to the way things were. I just need this anxiety to stop!" I began to realize the anxiety was pushing me into something that I'd never had to deal with.

My whole life I'd been pretty much in charge. I ran the Tom Lynch Show, even when it was crazy. When I did my thing, playing the outgoing entertainer, the charismatic priest, I got attention and was fun to be with. But I stayed on the surface and kept my relationships at a level I could handle. It had worked for a very long time.

This *something* that the anxiety was revealing was my own vulnerability – the realization that I couldn't control my life. I had been processing life with my own natural coping mechanisms and - a revelation even more frightening - the level of faith I'd been operating out of was not going to work anymore. It became clear that there's a thin line between living life to the fullest and being stuck in the Prison of Self for a life sentence.

I struggled. What was I going to do? Who was I becoming? My initial tendency was to redouble my efforts to get my life back in check. To work harder at being who I always was, with a few minor adjustments – in other words, put new wine into old wineskins. Tightening my grasp only brought me deeper into the Prison of Self. I grappled with this nagging question: *Do I stay on the surface of life or do I plunge deeper into the mystery of life and of God?* At times it seemed easier to go back to the Prison of Self, put on my uniform, listen to the internal loudspeaker, ruminate over clips of my past and fantasies of my future over and over. But, once awareness dawned, I knew I couldn't do that.

A voice resounded inside me: Live! Live! Don't die before you're dead! I knew if I went back I could survive in prison, but the hope of living a life of joy, peace, freedom, and love would fade until I became one of the walking dead. I began to realize that if I couldn't be vulnerable, I would never allow myself to be loved or be able to love at a deep level. That was a haunting insight. If I couldn't love at a deeper level, could I really minister to anyone in a meaningful way? How could I touch into anyone else's vulnerability if I couldn't get in touch with my own? These questions reflected the beginning of the dismantling of my ego self and of my naïve and reasonable faith.

MORTALITY

There was another major conversion experience in my life that forced me to confront, not only my vulnerability, but also my own mortality. Over time, I'd had a series of noncancerous tumors removed from my feet. I'd had eight or nine operations on my feet at that point, to remove tumors produced by a condition called fibromatosis – gangly tumors that grow like knotty tendrils producing painful lumps in the feet. I'd recently had another one – it had almost become routine.

I was alone at my desk in the Parish Center late that evening. The phone rang - my foot surgeon, Dr. Peter Blume. "Tom, Peter Blume. How're you doing? " I was struck by the fact that he called just to check in. We made a few moments of small talk and there was a short pause where he should have been saying *Take care, see you at your post-op appointment.* Instead, he cleared his throat. "As usual, we did a biopsy...you're aware that these tumors are almost never cancerous – but as a precaution..."

I heard him speaking but his words became strangely distant. I was startled. My heart began to race.

"...cancerous...a sarcoma...extremely rare...sent it on to Yale New Haven, then to Sloan Kettering. They're sorting through whether it's a "lazy" or an "aggressive" tumor." He paused. "Tom? "

"Yes..." I was nearly speechless for a moment – a real rarity. "Well, what does that mean? What happens now?" My voice didn't sound like my own.

"Let's set you up with an oncologist and a plastic surgeon, in case we need to operate."

"If it's aggressive – what are the options? "

"Well," he replied, "I don't think it's aggressive..."

"But if it is," I insisted, "the options? "

Another moment of silence. "Amputation. But let's not get ahead of ourselves. We need the test results first. If the tumor extends beyond the foot to various parts of the leg, you'll have to make a decision – but let's cross that bridge when we come to it."

I hung up. The word *cancer* whirled around in my head. I didn't want my foot or leg to be amputated. But cancer could spread. I'd suffer. Maybe I'd die. It hit me like cold water thrown in my face. Was I ready to die? I still had a life time ahead of me. I couldn't imagine it. It was surreal. The doctor's words hung around my neck like a heavy weight.

I limped, day by day, through the next two weeks, literally and figuratively. Ups and downs. The loudspeaker in the Prison of Self was driving me crazy – why…why…why…what if…what if… I couldn't concentrate on work, or even conversations. I became a zombie, muddling through my days, my ministry, my personal caretaking, my relationships.

My regular doctor called to reassure me. "Since the Vietnam War they've been doing great work on prosthetics for amputees." That did a lot to allay my fears. A few nights later, I was mindlessly losing myself in CNN and a report came on about the improvement of prosthetics for leg amputees. I said to myself, "Is the Lord trying to tell me something? Is He preparing me for my meeting with the oncologist?"

My sister Meggie accompanied me to my oncology appointment. There were a lot of patients waiting. I looked around – all of these people were in the cancer club. I desperately didn't want to belong. One by one they were called in, until my sister and I were the last ones in the waiting room. I'd started to sweat – was he purposely taking me at the very end of his day to deliver what would be devastating news? Trying for some levity, I leaned over to Meggie and said, "Maybe we should start planning the going away party for my leg." I tried to laugh, but it wasn't funny.

It turned out to be a lazy sarcoma and the margins were clear. I left the office, exhaled for what seemed to be the first time in weeks, said a prayer of thanks, and went out for dinner. At the restaurant I ordered a stiff drink, feeling as though I'd somehow dodged a bullet. For the first time, my mortality was staring me in the face. A nagging question crept into my head: Was my faith strong enough to freely embrace my *own* suffering and dying? It hadn't felt that way. Another chipping away – this time of an illusion I'd held about my own attitudes about living, and dying. What, I wondered, did it say about my faith?

Major Loss

Experiencing major losses also exacerbates this sense of our own mortality. I'd had many relatives pass away – older aunts and uncles, grandparents, the parents of my friends. When I was a kid, these deaths produced curiosity. As I got older it was often sad, but not earth-shattering. All of these deaths were comfortably distant.

However, when my own mother was diagnosed with colon cancer that had spread to the liver, it was different. The doctor gave her twelve months. She was relatively comfortable, so, as a family, we decided against any invasive treatment. Over the next twenty-two months she just sort of faded away, loss upon loss, becoming less and less mobile, losing weight until she finally died quietly. Death struck very close to home. It was real.

A year later, one of my brothers-in law, Danny, died of a sudden heart attack. He had just turned 50, was in incredible shape, worked out regularly.

If that wasn't enough, in another year's time, death delivered a third calling card. My sister Maureen. "I just got the call," she said. "Breast cancer." It was inflammatory breast cancer – a death sentence at that time. She lasted two and a half years. I presided at her funeral mass and walked with my family through it. Her passing made death even more real to me. It resonated powerfully after my near miss a few years earlier. She was just a year and a half older than me.

Conversion as Dismantling

Loss upon loss. I became more and more conscious of the costs of living, affected by not only the deaths of loved ones, but by other losses in my life. Shattered dreams of idealism, especially in regard to my priesthood and the brokenness of the church. The disappointments of changing relationships and friendships. I desperately wanted life to be as it had been, but also didn't want to be numb anymore. I was exhausted from the self-imposed demands of my schedule, and, at the same time, tired of skimming the surface of life. In short, I was literally sick of being in the Prison of Self.

But, facing an unknown future wrought with the possibility of even more loss was terrifying. Every time I approached the precipice of change my ego asserted itself, urging me back from the edge: *Listen, Tommy – I got you this far, didn't I? You want to risk everything – your security, life as you know it? You turn your back on what you know and you'll fall apart. Just hang on. Get a grip. You're strong enough, bold enough, brave enough, smart enough, and have enough resources to beat these things. Be the master of your own destiny! You've done it before, and you can do it again.*

I heard my ego speaking, but with my vulnerability, the loss of dreams and relationships, and faced with my own mortality, I began to question the validity of this inner voice that had been my cheerleader all along. The sense that I could control things on my own had been shattered like glass. I began to realize that everyone and everything I touched was broken. By not really dealing with my own vulnerability, mortality, and losses, I could see that when my turn to die came, I'd most certainly add great mental, emotional and spiritual suffering to whatever physical pain life had in store.

As a priest, I began to feel like a fraud. What did I truly believe? Where was the Good News, proclaimed by the Lord, in my preaching? In my life? Did I really believe it? After all I'd been through, had I still been completely co-opted by the culture, believing that life was really all about self reliance rooted in success, achievement, competition, productivity? My training in the seminary did not prepare me for this. I found I had few practical skills for applying what the Gospels taught in life-giving ways. The message I got about the mysteries of suffering and loss was to simply "offer it up" – what I saw at the time as the spiritual equivalent of "sucking it up."

I became acutely aware that if I couldn't face my *own* vulnerability, mortality, and losses, I surely wouldn't be able to help anyone else deal with theirs. My care and ministry for others would hollow out. I'd be going through the motions, but my spirit, passion, and commitment would die. To have given up wife and children to become a cynical old priest would be devastating – a waste of a life.

Without a doubt, academics or theology couldn't put the broken pieces of my ego, my beliefs, or my faith back together. I had changed, but persisted in clinging to the same old behaviors that could no longer sustain me. As Jesus said, you can't put new wine in old wine skins. I'd been confronted with my own weakness, been **dismantled.** I stood in darkness, broken, frightened, yet there was a dim flicker of hope - a generative pulsation hinting that these experiences *meant something* – something I still could not discern.

BEGINNING TO BREAK FREE FROM THE PRISON OF SELF - ACCEPTANCE

Gradually, after many stops and starts, I began to accept the brokenness of my life, facing my losses, embracing my vulnerabilities, and getting in touch with my own mortality. I stopped fighting against and running from these realities, and began to admit that what had been, would be no more. In other words, I started to relinquish control, to examine my priorities, and in doing so began to look at my life differently. I had to allow myself to grieve over my losses, reconcile with those I'd hurt or been hurt by. I was forced to acknowledge that I'd been compromising my health, and that I'd need to make some serious changes. I was not invincible after all. Little by little I began to experience a tentative kind of peace, while at the same time sensing an undercurrent of unrest – feeling the creative tension between the cultural values that had shaped me and my disillusionment with them.

This is not to suggest that I'd become comfortable with my situation. I hadn't. It seemed that with each subsequent trauma I found myself, once again, on the Path of Suffering, reluctantly adjusting to a "new normal." I would have done anything to go back to the mindless busyness

I'd become accustomed to. But, I knew that was impossible. I had to *accept* that my old values and aspirations had not served me well, nor would they save me from having to deal with the even greater losses that would surely come.

Acceptance – I knew I'd have to acknowledge and grapple with each "new normal." Redefine my relationships, my work, and self-image in a way that was, at the same time, more realistic and more forgiving. This gentle realism might allow me a greater degree of freedom. My agenda would be less driven, my priorities clearer. I'd need to use my time more selectively, with activities and relationships that were healthier. I'd try to increase my prayer life, exercise more, eat better, spend quality time with people who cared. I made an effort to do this, and my life improved. My anxiety decreased.

But, why then, was there still an undercurrent of tension beneath the surface of my life? I'd seen the same dynamic with people suffering from a serious or terminal illness. They'd fought their way through denial, became resigned to the reality before them, and gradually moved toward the more peaceful state of *acceptance*. They wanted to make the best use of their time, prioritize their relationships, and keep anxiety and sadness at a minimum. Enjoy what they could. From time to time, like me, they'd fall back into fear, regret, and worry – the by-products of *control*. While I'd been forced to admit that I could no longer keep all the balls in the air, I was still hanging on to some degree, manipulating things as much as I could. My focus continued to be ego-centered. I hadn't been able to make meaning of my suffering. Perhaps in more subtle ways, I was still struggling to control mystery rather than to stand in awe of it.

On my better days I told myself that the tension I felt was the foreshadowing of a new understanding of life pulling me closer to some as yet unimagined but more meaningful reality *beyond acceptance*. I found myself teetering on the edge of what felt like a dangerous cliff, knowing I had to somehow liberate myself from the shackles that held me. I clung to the edge for a long time. I knew I had to take a huge leap of faith.

But I wasn't quite ready yet.

CHAPTER 10

The Way of the Cross

IT WAS A cold, damp Friday night. I headed over to church to pray the Stations of the Cross – always one of my favorite devotions. The ritual was developed by Saint Francis of Assisi to help Christians who were unable to go to the Holy Land so that they could walk the journey of Jesus during his suffering, dying, and death.

The prevailing slump I was in made doing things, even things I'd always found life-giving, an effort. Sighing, I put on the vestments, lit the candles. In the dim light of the church each bronze plaque seemed to glow, drawing me toward the familiarity of the story we were about to commemorate once again.

I moved toward the first station, opening the book to the well-known text. Through the years, I'd read the words so often I sometimes missed their impact. In times of stress, times of tension and transition, it was even easier to read without comprehension or real emotional investment - drawn to the words, and yet somehow not willing to touch into them.

The acolyte carried the cross and set it before the first station. The candle-bearer beside him looked to me expectantly. I felt restless, anxious. I needed to find a way to focus. To get out of my own way. Without consciously deciding to do so, I placed myself in the shoes (or sandals) of Jesus – Jesus, the *man*. What would it have been like to walk his walk? This was my train of thought as I began the service.

"Please stand... The Son of Man must suffer greatly and be rejected by the elders, the chief priests, the scribes, and be killed and on the third day be raised. If anyone wishes to come after me he must deny himself and take up his cross daily and follow me. Whoever wishes to save his life will lose it, but whoever loses his life for my sake will save it."

THE FIRST STATION – PILATE CONDEMNS JESUS TO DEATH.

Jesus is handed over to Pilate to be condemned to death. His friends have betrayed, denied, and abandoned him. He is left alone to embrace the darkness of the moment. The soldiers have beaten him, and he is unfairly judged. Jesus is condemned to die a cruel and painful death - even though he is innocent of any crime.

Unfair – what was happening signaled the end of life as Jesus knew it. His life had turned on a dime. No going back. My heart stirred. I began to sweat. I was suddenly alert. This was a theme I could relate to. He had to deal with something thrust upon him that touched into his vulnerabilities and forced him to look death in the eye – to face something he'd prefer not to face.

THE SECOND STATION – JESUS TAKES UP HIS CROSS

Jesus opens his arms and takes up his cross, knowing full well the pain and agony lying ahead. He accepts his destiny even though he isn't guilty. It is unfair. Unjust. He does not deserve this fate imposed upon him.

As I read, I felt an empathy I'd never experienced before. When considering Jesus as a deity it had been easy to see him as above it all, able to take the condemnation, disappointment, fear, and regret in stride. After all, this was part of his Father's divine plan, wasn't it?

But, wouldn't Jesus the *man* have experienced what all human beings would feel? Walking in his footsteps I could hear him lament, "Why me? Can this cup pass me by? Do I trust in God my Father or do I trust myself to somehow get things back in control again? " Brought to a dark precipice, he had to make a decision – either to enter this pit of darkness, or to walk away, fight the inevitable and cling to the past, or surrender to it.

Reading the words, my own vulnerability, the losses I'd experienced, and the awareness of my mortality resonated powerfully. Maybe I was seeing the ramifications clearly for the first time. Letting go of how I defined my life, my dreams, my attachments meant that life as I knew it would be no more. Continuing on this walk with Jesus would mean taking a huge leap of faith. I would have to die to myself and embrace my crosses. It would mean free-falling without the benefit of a safety net. Trading the known for the mystery of whatever might be next.

I thought of the words of author Dr. Gerald May: "If we really knew what we are called to relinquish on this journey, our defenses would never allow us to take the first step. Sometimes the only way we can enter the deeper dimensions of the journey is by being unable to see where we're going."

I felt the weight of each step as I walked toward the third station. Lost in my own thoughts, I almost failed to notice one of my long-time parishioners seated at the end of the pew. Her husband George sat beside her, eyes closed, holding her hand. I knew Sonia's story. She'd suffered from breast cancer – had been in remission for a little over five years. And then, just when she thought she was safe, she had a recurrence...

THE THIRD STATION – JESUS FALLS THE FIRST TIME.

Under the weight of the cross, in his weakened physical state, Jesus stumbles and falls. He lies there in the dust at the soldiers' feet. People mock him and scream for him to get up. The pain from the scourging and the crown of thorns is excruciating. He finds it nearly impossible to move, yet somehow he rises and walks on.

Sonia's gaze met mine. Then she looked away, dabbed at her eyes with a shredded tissue. She seemed tired, spent. I understood, suddenly, that she was seeing what I saw – but that she comprehended, far better than I, what Jesus had been feeling – because she was living it along with him.

She'd been condemned with a diagnosis, she received her cross. She'd walked in faith and optimism, believing she was going to beat the disease. It had been tough, but she'd been able to maintain her commitments, her work, her family life. She'd become an advocate, spokeswoman and inspiration for breast cancer survivors. Women looked up to her, credited her with instilling them with hope, with strength. And now...

THE FOURTH STATION – JESUS MEETS HIS MOTHER.

Mary, the mother of Jesus, who cared for him so tenderly during his early years, sees her son being led to execution. Grief-stricken, she watches. There is nothing she can do but stand beside him, offering love and support. Seeing his mother suffering causes Jesus even greater emotional pain. All they can do is look at each other in love. Knowing she is there in his darkest hour gives Jesus strength.

Station to station, the words continued to jump off the page. Jesus, comforted by his mother *and* comforting her. Family helping family, as best they could. Sometimes just being there was really all that was possible. Even in their pain, they accepted and extended love to the other. Sonia and George, side by side, their individual and shared pain, anxieties, losses intertwined, walking the same path. No one suffers alone. Always the tension of accepting help or pushing it away.

What, I wondered, did Jesus feel as he moved toward the fifth and sixth stations? What did Sonia feel? And, in my own small troubling life, I found myself asking if anyone would really ever love and care for me... and if so, could I accept it graciously, lovingly?

THE FIFTH STATION – JESUS IS HELPED BY SIMON.

As he continues to carry his cross Jesus grows weaker. It's possible he could die before reaching his place of crucifixion. His captors press an onlooker named Simon into service, to help support the weight of the cross and ease Jesus' burden.

I thought of the medical staff who'd cared for me during all the surgeries on my feet - who would have strived to help me adjust to life as an amputee if it had come to that. Sometimes the easiest care to accept comes from outside sources – strangers, in fact – the special nurses, aides, doctors, therapists who've stood with us in kindness without being overcome by anxiety and sadness. Sonia's doctor, who was always just a phone call away, could calm her fears in an objective but kind way – something overprotective family and friends might be unable to do.

THE SIXTH STATION – VERONICA WIPES THE FACE OF JESUS.

Jesus' face is bruised and swollen, caked in blood, sweat, and dirt. Despite warnings from his captors, Veronica, moved with pity, emerges from the crowd and gently wipes his face. Jesus graciously accepts her care.

During times of challenge, the parish family reached out, sending meals, providing transport, and performing household chores for Sonia and George, but their prayers were even more powerful. As Sonia's world diminished, the faith community reminded her that she was part of a bigger story – not only as a member of our church, but, more importantly, as a part of the body of Christ. On days when the ravages of illness tried her faith, the community was there as a reminder of what we believe – that God's presence in the world is with us, in us, and for us, even in our darkest moments. Likewise, Sonia was a living testament of faith to those who ministered to her. I thought of my friends, Fr. Carl Arico and Fr. Tom Boland, the strength of their belief supporting me through the years - reminding me to trust God, validating the faith that I sometimes lost sight of.

SEVENTH STATION – JESUS FALLS A SECOND TIME.

As Jesus continues on the road to Calvary his emotional pain and multiple injuries further weaken and discourage him. Despite the love and care he's received, he is overcome by a sense of utter despair and debilitating loss, and collapses, again, under the weight of it.

Even though Jesus allowed himself to give and receive love during each step of his journey, even though he was cared for by family and others, the emotional energy that it took to deal with suffering and pain had wearied him. Like all of us who struggle, he fell beneath the burden. I thought of my own ongoing feelings of discontent, my unwillingness to really be open to change, despite the encouragement and validation of others in my life. And Sonia, suffering a recurrence that involved even greater loss than she experienced during the first phase of her disease, the realization that there was probably no going back, that the path she was on would be long and grueling and would lead her to only *greater* pain and loss – it was easy to see how she would fall under the tremendous weightiness of the situation. She had told me of nights lying awake, the darkness looming endlessly before her, crying out to her God, "I just can't continue to go on like this..." The utter aloneness of it.

Falling under the weight of the cross. The question at this crossroads is - do I accept this descent into the darkness of the unknown in a spirit of acceptance and freedom? Or do I continue to fight the un-fightable, giving away whatever days I have left? In essence, do I choose to die before I'm dead?

EIGHTH STATION – JESUS MEETS THE WOMEN OF JERUSALEM.

The women and children watching Jesus struggle are stricken with grief and sadness. It is difficult to watch someone suffer and feel powerless to alter the course of events. Realizing that they too will someday have to face great loss, and take a final walk toward death alone, Jesus tells them to pray for themselves and for their children.

I see that there is a point at which we have to descend into the abyss, into the unknown, *alone*. Others may feel for us, but while their compassion and empathy is appreciated, each and every one of us has to walk this walk on our own – it's the common cross of all humanity. *Weep for yourselves and for your children – what I need from you is not your grief – I need a reminder from you that God is with me.* Jesus needs to detach from the lamenting women – carrying his own pain along with theirs only adds weight to the cross and prevents him from moving forward. Unbridled grief prevents the person suffering from embracing their destiny. How much, I wondered, did Sonia fight a battle she couldn't win, in order to give those around her hope? To play the role they needed her to play – a role in which she could somehow conquer the unconquerable and save them from *their* pain at her impending death.

In my own journey, I thought of how often friends, family, parishioners, and colleagues strove to maintain the status quo. They accepted me as long as I didn't change in any way and push them out of their comfort zones. Resistance became the dynamic of these relationships – a painful situation for all concerned. How threatening and confusing it can be for those around us when we let go of who we've been in order to emerge as a new, and yet unknown, creation.

NINTH STATION – JESUS FALLS A THIRD TIME.

Overwhelming physical and emotional pain, and the losses that go with it lead Jesus into a state of spiritual desolation. His faith is shaken. He wonders if God has abandoned him. Realizing there is no relief ahead of him, and no way back, he feels he simply cannot go on. Exhausted, helpless, he falls a third time.

Walking alone isn't easy. This is the final wrestling between trusting God and trusting self, and the last attempt to maintain control and a belief in your own ability to cope and survive. Each step is harder than the one before. You hit the ground and realize with certainty, perhaps for the first time, that you will not overcome this challenge. We realize we are no longer in control; in fact, we are helpless. There is a strange relief in this. As author Gerald May has written: "When we cannot chart our own course, we become vulnerable to God's protection, and the darkness becomes a "guiding night," a "night more kindly than the dawn." I think of Sonia saying what had become her mantra, "It's okay…God is good…" A faith born of suffering.

TENTH STATION - JESUS IS STRIPPED OF HIS GARMENTS.

Somehow Jesus has finally arrived at Golgotha, to the top of the hill where he is to be crucified. The soldiers strip him of his garments, exposing him to the crowd. He is reduced to nothing, robbed of his dignity and identity. Onlookers jeer – "So this is the King of the Jews!"

What were Sonia's garments – the roles and titles she clothed herself in? Her position at the University and her community there – stripped away. A cancer survivor – stripped away. An outspoken advocate and symbol of hope for women with cancer – stripped away. An involved mother and wife – stripped away. An independent woman – stripped away. Everything close to the heart, all the strivings, the longings, ripped from her. Each causes a rupture, and oh, how we bleed. *Who am I now?* we wonder, as this hemorrhage leaves us drowning in a deep depression.

Who would I be, if not priest, pastor, counselor, preacher? Could it be that the "me" God loves is *none* of these things that I cling to so desperately? That what God loves is the *essence* of the spirit hidden beneath all the rest? Regardless, in our humanness, we grieve over the stripping away of our false self, and cling to it as long as we can.

ELEVENTH STATION – JESUS IS NAILED TO HIS CROSS.

The executioners stretch Jesus on the cross and drive nails into his hands and feet. Why, Jesus wonders, can't I just die already? Why do I have to continue to suffer like this? The cross is hoisted and the vigil begins. Darkness descends.

No hope of return. In fact, the pain of the present moment is such that any yearning for life as it was dissipates, replaced by a longing for death – death as a release from what *is*. Sonia wasn't quite there yet. True, the neuropathy in her hands and feet, the pain that came with each inhalation, the wracking cough, never-ending treatments, the pervasive fatigue and weakness, a heaviness that hung over her like she never experienced before - all of this pulled her closer and closer to this critical transition in which we know, at the core of who we are, not only that there's no going back, but we no longer want to. The realization dawns that, like Jesus, we're nailed to our suffering. We cannot run from it. We cannot fight it. There's no escape. We have to hang there in it, and be transformed by it.

And what about me? Did my current situation hurt badly enough for me to relinquish it for something else? Understanding dawned, looking at Sonia, that going back to business as usual was no longer an option.

110

I would have to die to what was, venture into the mystery of unknowing, and trust that something better would emerge.

TWELFTH STATION...JESUS DIES ON THE CROSS.

Jesus hangs on the cross for three endless hours. Some of the women keep vigil. The fickle crowd jeers. They scream for him to come down, to save himself. He is clearly not the Messiah they had hoped he would be. His disciples desert him. The soldiers pierce his side with a lance, cast lots for his clothes. Most pass by, shake their heads, and continue on with their lives. Before he dies he calls out, "Father, forgive them for they know not what they do. It is finished." Then he surrenders his spirit and dies.

How, I wondered, was Jesus able to trust so radically, to die in such a loving stance? Can any of us grasp what it takes to submit to the unknown? Is it born of strength or of weakness? Is it a giving up or a letting go? Is it the end, or the beginning of something new?

I considered this as I inched toward the decision about whether or not to surrender to whatever death I'd need to face in order to emerge, a new creation. I glanced again at Sonia. Eyes closed. Was she wondering the same thing?

THIRTEENTH STATION...JESUS IS TAKEN DOWN FROM THE CROSS.

Mary Magdalene and Mary, the mother of James of Joses, watch from a distance, overwhelmed with grief and loss, but relieved that his suffering is finally over. Joseph of Arimathea removes the body of Jesus, and along with Nicodemus, anoints him with a mixture of myrrh and aloes. They bind his body in linen according to Jewish burial customs.

Who, I wondered, would stand with me through the unknown changes ahead? Would I be embraced on the other side of transformation, or forgotten, left behind? Did I believe what Jesus taught enough to surrender to it? And, I wondered, if I couldn't allow myself to let go, to die to self in this relatively small way, how would I ever be able to enter into my actual, physical death in a spirit of freedom and hope?

FOURTEENTH STATION...JESUS IS PLACED IN THE TOMB.

Joseph of Arimathea lays the body of Jesus into a new tomb, hewn out of rock. Then, he rolls a large stone against the entrance. Mary Magdalene and the other Mary sit, opposite the grave. Gradually the mourners leave, in grief and silence.

I tried to keep in mind that the journey continues. That Holy Week doesn't stop at Good Friday. The feeling that all was lost continued to nag at me, that life as I knew it was over, yet there was no clear sense of what would be birthed from this death. This would be a resting time, waiting in darkness for whatever dawn was to come. I was in a tomb of sorts, keeping vigil in the wake of loss. I needed time to adjust to the dark, to begin to see and hear things in a new way, to respond differently to life. Instead of cold fear or hot anger, instead of overwhelming sadness or anxiety, I began to feel the faintest stirrings of hope.

Think about the times when your life turned on a dime – when you experienced loss, were forced to let go, to accept changes you would have preferred not to embrace. Didn't the evolution of that experience mirror the way of the Cross – feeling condemned, taking up the cross, falling under its weight – once, twice, three times - being stripped of all that matters? Being nailed to your suffering?

Usually, while struggling through loss (whether the loss of a job, a dream, a relationship, health, or the actual process of physical dying and death) it's difficult to see the forest for the trees. In other words, it

112

can be nearly impossible to recognize the basic over-arching movement that's taking place.

It was suddenly so clear to me: While we'll all have to walk this ultimate path, none of us - not me, not Sonia, and not you – have to venture out without a guide. Jesus said, *"I am the way, the truth, and the life..."* I'd always looked at the Passion of Christ in isolation – as a uniquely painful *exception* to the normal human experience. However, walking the Stations of the Cross alongside Sonia, in the context of my own struggles, brought me an important insight – that suffering, loss, and surrender *is the normal path we all will take.* Jesus, the man, walked the Path of Suffering, validating our humanity, experiencing the range of emotions, hopes, and fears that we all will ultimately have to face. Jesus, too, recognized and anticipated the pain he was going to go through. Like all of us, he would have preferred to avoid this path of pain and suffering.

But, at the same time, he knew all was not lost. Jesus knew where his strength came from – that it was God's strength that carried him through it. He was standing in a transformative moment in which his heart was open to a mystery greater than himself.

The late Joseph Campbell, scholar, mythologist, and writer, spoke of this alternate consciousness of Jesus that can transform the suffering of the path into something greater, something more life-giving and meaningful:

"We have not even to risk the adventure alone, for the heroes of all time have gone before us — the labyrinth is thoroughly known. We have only to follow the thread of the hero path, and where we had thought to find an abomination, we shall find a god; where we had thought to slay another, we shall slay ourselves; where we had thought to travel outward, we shall come to the center of our own existence. And where we had thought to be alone, we shall be with all the world."

We may see our tragic situation or illness as an abomination, but some, in and through the experience, instead discover God. As most attempt to travel outward, to run from the situation, a few move inward, to the core of who they are, where God abides.

CHAPTER 11

The Indwelling of God

THINK ABOUT THOSE times in your life you'd prefer to forget. Painful, stressful times that challenged you in ways you never thought you could withstand. How often have you reflected back and wondered, "How did I ever get through it? "

Good question.

We somehow muddle along in the darkness, hands extended, hanging on, groping, feeling our way on instinct (or adrenalin) alone. And then we seem, at some point, to stumble into the light. Did we accomplish this ourselves?

Barbara received an insight into this while doing some online research. Quite by accident she came across something called "The Ruby Slippers Principle."

In *The Wizard of Oz*, Dorothy asks Glinda the Good Witch, "Oh, will you help me? Can you help me?" Glinda tells her that she doesn't need to be helped any longer. That she's always had the power to go back to Kansas. Irritated by this, the Scarecrow asks Glinda, "Then why didn't you tell her before?" Glinda responds, "Because she wouldn't have believed me. She had to learn it for herself." Rather than asking how to get what she wanted, perhaps Dorothy should have been asking, "How do I recognize what I already have?"

So many people I've visited who are struggling in a difficult situation, suffering from a serious loss or illness, or standing in the throes of the dying process, have told their own version of Dorothy's "Ruby Slippers Principle."

Elise had suffered from lupus for more than 30 years. The disease had progressed to the point where it was affecting her organs. When I entered the room she was barely able to lift her hand to wave.

"How are you doing, Elise? " I asked. She sighed and shook her head.

"Father, it's funny," she said. "I'm so weak, most days I can't do anything. I don't know how I manage to get through it. My friends and family all say, 'I can't believe how strong you are.' Strong?" She laughed - a sound with little humor in it. "I'm not strong at all. It all comes from here..." She tapped her fingers on her chest.

"What's that? " I asked.

"What keeps me going... "

I looked at her, eyebrows raised.

"You know, Father," she replied, "God. It's God that keeps me going." She smiled wryly. "Didn't know I had it in me..."

Most of us don't...

THE MYTH OF SELF

It's easiest to recognize the "Ruby Slippers" phenomena following difficult or tragic moments. Though we're more open to seeing this dynamic in the aftermath of some trauma, the same power that propelled us through that difficulty is available to us every day of our lives – but we don't really believe it. Nor do we want to acknowledge that we need it.

We've been conditioned to think we should be able to handle whatever life throws our way. That we can pull ourselves up by our own bootstraps. How many times have you heard TV self-help gurus talk about how we need to *love* ourselves, *forgive* ourselves, *heal* ourselves in order to survive the tough stuff? If it was as easy as that, why wouldn't we all just love, forgive, and heal ourselves into a sense of fullness, enlightenment, and peace and be done with it?

This "myth of the self" actually does more harm than good, because when we're told we must love, forgive, and heal ourselves and we can't seem to do it, we experience a sense of failure on top of the inherent challenges of the situation. We're dealt a double blow – not only are we feeling unlovable, hurt, and guilty, but our self-worth, self-esteem, and self-respect have tanked. In fact, we can no more love, forgive, and heal ourselves than we can raise ourselves from the dead. For this, we need to look to something greater than ourselves. Without looking to this higher power we're likely to struggle and strive on our own, only to fall short. And when this happens, where do we end up? Right back in the Prison of Self.

Can it be that when we've found ourselves on the other side of darkness, we actually survived *in spite of* our frail attempts to control the situation? That we'd unconsciously drawn from some higher power? That we unknowingly accessed the same source of strength that allowed Jesus to walk the Stations of the Cross in a stance of love, forgiveness, nonviolence, and faith? Think about it. What's more likely? That we mustered up some miraculous super-human strength and finally got a grip on the situation, or that when we absolutely couldn't continue another day, another step, another moment under our own power, we let go...and something greater than all of it took hold and carried us through? A *savior*, perhaps?

JESUS' SOURCE OF STRENGTH

I contemplated all of this as I looked at Jesus, the man, and asked myself, "What exactly empowered him to walk the stations of his suffering, dying, and death?" How did Jesus consistently respond in love throughout these outrageously difficult and painful circumstances? Could he do this because he was both human and divine – that his divinity afforded him a level of strength unavailable to us mere mortals? Was he able to love, forgive, and heal *himself* through it? Or was he endowed by a reservoir of strength within him that he drew from?

We get a sense of this from the following excerpt from Lamentations 3:17-26:

My soul is deprived of peace, I have forgotten what happiness is;
I tell myself my future is lost, all that I had hoped from the Lord.
The thought of my homeless poverty is wormwood and gall;
Remembering it over and over leaves my soul downcast within me.
But I will call this to mind, as my reason to have hope:
The favors of the Lord are not exhausted,
His mercies are not spent; They are renewed each morning, so great is his
faithfulness.
My portion is the Lord, says my soul;
Therefore will I hope in him. Good is the Lord to the one who waits for him,
To the soul that seeks him; It is good to hope in silence for the saving help
of the Lord.

How was it that Jesus accessed this hope, and is it something we can access as well?

With these questions in mind I revisited the Scriptures, searching for some insight. As I began reading the Gospels, I became aware of some passages in which Jesus withdrew into solitude, far from the crowds, away from his disciples. He would retreat in order to spend time in prayer and reflection. Acutely aware of the presence of God, Jesus tapped into it often and nurtured this intimate connection. It's also clear that Jesus experienced this intimacy as a oneness with God.

In John 14:10, Jesus asked his disciples: *"Do you not believe that I am in the Father and the Father is in me? "* And in Verse 11: *"Believe me when I say that I am in the Father and the Father is in me."* In Verse 20: *On that day you will realize that I am in my Father and you are in me and I in you.*

This indwelling of God was clearly Jesus' saving source of mercy and hope, offering him the love and healing that none of us can provide for ourselves. His oneness with his Father didn't spare Jesus his passion, suffering, and death – none of us can escape that. But it did enable him to move through it in hope, peace, joy, and love.

THE INDWELLING OF GOD – THE INCARNATION

The church refers to this indwelling of God as the *Incarnation*. Most Christians, on an intellectual level, accept the idea that God's presence is manifested in the universe, in our world, in the person of Jesus Christ, in the celebration of the Sacraments, and, to some extent, in the presence of the Holy Spirit within each person. But, even when we profess to believe this, we tend to think of God as being some abstract force "out there somewhere." As a boy I was taught that God was present on the altar, in the tabernacle, and in heaven. We often talk about someone who's died as having "gone to heaven" – that faraway place up in the sky where God resides.

These ideas, and the images and language we use to represent them all imply *separation from God*. So, it's no wonder we have difficulty believing that God is a living presence and source of strength within us that can be accessed and experienced firsthand. For most of us who have not matured past the stages of Naïve and/or Reasonable faith, who feel we must earn or bargain for God's love, that sense of separation is even greater. We feel that in order to discover God we must search far and wide and multiply many prayers and good works. The focus is on finding God outside of ourselves rather than discovering God within. This is sometimes called the "God and me" mentality – again, pointing toward distance rather than oneness.

In his book, *The Dark Night of the Soul*, Dr. Gerald May articulates this:

As soon as we use the label "God" or "divine presence" we make an object of it, separate from ourselves. Taken together, these reasons encourage us to dwell in the more comfortable, controllable world of "God and me," rather than the vague, vulnerable realm of "God in me and I in God." Clinging to the "God and me" mentality, we actually come to believe such bogus sayings as "God helps those who help themselves" or "Pray as if everything depended on God, but work as if everything depended on yourself."

Likewise, Fr. Thomas Keating said:

The beginning of the spiritual journey is the realization; not just the information, but a real interior conviction that there is a higher power, or God. Or to make it as easy as possible for everyone, there is an Other: capital O. The second step is to try and become the Other: still a capital O. And finally the realization that there is no other. You and the other are One: always have been, always will be. You just think that you aren't.

WHY IS THIS IDEA SO DIFFICULT TO EMBRACE?

It's clear that most of us hold the "God out there" view. Think about it – if we *really* believed that God dwelled within each and every one of us, would we continue to exhibit the kind of blatant disregard we often have for others? Would we be so easily able to judge others and cast them aside as "bad" or "worthless"? Would we amass resources when every minute another 15 people in this world die of starvation? Would we continue to be as hard on ourselves as we are, as unforgiving and self-loathing as we tend to be?

The implications of truly believing in the incarnation are huge. If we really believed it we'd relate to ourselves and others very differently.

If we actually accepted that God dwelled within us we'd approach our own sickness, dying, and death with less trepidation and sadness, and with greater faith, hope, and love.

HUNGER AND THIRST FOR GOD

But are we really ever far from our innate desire to experience our one-ness with God? I believe that, unconsciously, we spend our entire lives searching for what is already there. *We just displace and misname the object of our search.*

Just look around at the sense of vague discontent that seems almost epidemic in our society. The compulsive need to strive, accomplish, achieve, excel, obtain, amass... it drives us to fill every minute of every day with intense busy-ness and anxiety. A better job, a bigger house, travel, the right car, clothes, toys, relationships...the objects of our long-ings seem endless. So often, once the object of our effort is realized, the satisfaction we feel is fleeting. We're immediately filled with even greater longings, more challenging goals, steeper expectations, the objects of which become harder to obtain. The pattern repeats, and repeats, and repeats. We continue to endeavor for things that fail to fulfill us.

Could it be that what we've been thrashing about for is really God? That this is precisely why we can never seem to fill the insatiable space inside us? As St. Augustine said, "You have made us for yourself, O Lord, and our heart is restless until it rests in you." Perhaps, like Dorothy, we're searching for something we've had all along - we just haven't figured out how to open the gift.

No matter how much we live outside ourselves chasing after this or that, intuitively we know that God is waiting for us to turn around, get off the surface and plunge into the mystery of God's presence within us. This poem, by 13th - century Sufi mystic and poet, Rumi, expresses it beautifully – how patient God is, how God views our misguided pursuits through eyes of understanding and love.

It's Rigged

It's rigged—everything in your favor,
So there is nothing to worry about.
Is there some position you want,
Some office, some award, some con, some lover,
Maybe two, maybe three, maybe four – all at once,
Maybe a relationship with God?
I know there is a gold mine in you, when you find it
The wonderment of the earth's gifts you will lay
Aside as naturally as does
a child a doll.
But, dear, how sweet you look to me kissing the unreal;
Comfort, fulfill yourself in any way possible—
do that until you ache, until you ache,
then come to me again.
(translation: Daniel Ladinsky, used with permission)

Regardless of our worldly focus, we will all eventually become aware of our oneness with God. For a few, this happens during the "green times" of life. For many more, it happens when tragedy strikes, as our Naïve and Reasonable Faith become dismantled and a new consciousness of God is revealed. For a time, we all fight to hold onto our independence and resist relinquishing control. Some will fight right to the end. Regardless of our willingness or lack of it, one way or another, we all will recognize that we've been one with God all along.

Think of it like this--a set of toddler twins is exhausted. It's been a long, full day and it's time for bed. One child resists, throws a tantrum, asks for glass after glass of water, screams when the parent tries to tuck him in. Climbs out of the crib until he finally cries himself to sleep on the floor, exhausted and spent. The other twin allows himself to be read to, snuggles up next to mom, and drifts off to sleep. Both children will eventually rest, safe and sound, recipients of the loving care of their parents. But the journey to that peaceful place for each of them is very different.

This is how it is for all of us. We will all, eventually, on this side of the grave or the other, become aware of our oneness with God and rest peacefully in it. For some it will be a journey marked with resistance, anger, fear, anxiety, regret, and sadness. Others will experience the journey as bittersweet, perhaps, at times, uncomfortable, but the underlying current on which they travel is made of trust, love, peace, gratitude, and hope.

The good news is we don't have to "do it right". Just as the parent who watches the resistant toddler screaming his way to bed knows that at the end of the day this beloved, headstrong child will rest, God walks with a dying loved one who spends the last chapter of life fighting the un-fightable, knowing that regardless of his stance, he will ultimately be embraced by God.

An ever-deepening awareness of God's indwelling can change the nature of our final journey. Experiencing a sense of oneness with our Creator can lead us to discover a new and life-giving way to walk this path.

CHAPTER 12

A New Way of Walking the Path

"Everything can be taken from a man but one thing --
the last of the human freedoms -- to choose one's
attitude in any given set of circumstances, to choose
one's own way."

-- VIKTOR FRANKL, FROM HIS BOOK *MAN'S SEARCH FOR
MEANING*

DURING THE SECOND World War, Frankl, a well-known psychiatrist of Jewish heritage, found himself a prisoner in the Nazi concentration camps in Hitler's Germany. During his internment he lost his parents and his brother, as well as his pregnant wife. While others became depressed, suicidal, bitter, overwhelmed with fear and anxiety, Frankl was able to somehow see the situation through a different lens. Instead of viewing his circumstances at face value, he was able to place his experiences in the context of a broader reality, to believe that from his hardships he could, if he was willing, discern and embrace some deeper meaning and value to, what for others, was simply tragedy.

How was he able to do this?

Frankl held the conviction that his life – every aspect of it - *meant something.* And that once a person recognized his or her purpose, when one knew the 'why' of their existence, they could almost always bear the 'how.'

Of course, Jesus, during his Passion, is a prime example of the 'why' making the 'how' bearable. There are other examples of this – Ghandi and Martin Luther King, Jr. - tolerating terrible abuse because they were devoted to a greater cause that gave their suffering (and their dying) meaning.

The question we ordinary people may be asking is, "Yes, but where is the greater meaning in *my* life?" We certainly don't see ourselves as the Savior of the World, or as someone with the compassion and courage to survive a concentration camp, or possessing the charism, boldness, and vision to lead a nation in a movement of nonviolent civil disobedience. Most of us are just regular people living rather mundane lives. So, when life turns on a dime, where is the meaning? What is the point? How can we make significance of this path toward sickness, dying and death?

HOW TO WALK THE PATH – THE CHOICE IS YOURS

While the physical experience of the body breaking down is ultimately unavoidable, the *way* we move along the path from dying to death can change everything. If we choose to look at the breaking down of our bodies as *only* a tragic sequence of events it *can* seem meaningless. Then the only way to react is to redouble our efforts to control the uncontrollable. Remember - when the fulcrum tips in this direction and our life is dominated by control, it's impossible to extend love to even those closest to us. Those around you can only be viewed in terms of what they're doing or not doing for you – and you begin to lose your capacity to love. Your world shrinks, isolation and loneliness become the norm, which intensifies your emotional, mental, and spiritual suffering.

There are also ways to bolster the natural coping mechanisms – the use of drugs to calm anxiety and fear can provide physical relief, but without being accompanied by the internal spiritual work of letting go can numb the emotions and hamper the work that can serve to liberate you and your loved ones during this process.

If you choose to address this superficially, dealing primarily with the challenges of your losses and/or disease, you'll likely have little energy left for anything else. In addition, you might experience a persistent, uneasy feeling that you could spend the last of your days suffering as a captive in the Prison of Self. It's one reason why people who often seemed unhappy during life continue to strive for still more days – because they've never realized what it is to have been free.

The other implication of this is even more important – *the sense that choosing to traverse this path differently might just be the key to finally escape from prison and attain a freedom you've never known before.* What if this tragedy is actually a unique opportunity for grace, for enlightenment, for freedom – to experience a much higher level of consciousness that will allow you to see through the same lens Viktor Frankl did? This is a prospect that cannot be realized without a huge leap of faith. The Prophet Isaiah speaks of what those who choose to travel this final path at a deeper level can experience:

> *They will see the glory of the Lord, the splendor of our God. Strengthen the hands that are feeble, make firm the knees that are weak, say to those whose hearts are frightened: be strong, fear not! Here is your God, he comes with vindication; with divine recompense he comes to save you. Then will the eyes of the blind be opened, the ears of the deaf be cleared; then will the lame leap like a stag, then the tongue of the dumb shall sing. Streams will burst forth in the desert, and rivers in the steppe. The burning sands will become pools, and the thirsty ground, springs of water; the abode where jackals lurch will be a marsh for the reed and papyrus. A highway will be there, called the holy way; No one unclean may pass over it, nor fools go astray on it. No lion will be there, nor beast of prey go up to be met upon it. It is for those with a journey to make, and on it the redeemed will walk. Those whom the Lord has ransomed will return and enter Zion singing, crowned with everlasting joy; They will meet with joy and gladness, sorrow and mourning will flee.* (Isaiah 35: 1-10)

This is an understanding not unique to the Judeo Christian faith. The following Buddhist saying captures the same truth: *Suffering, if it does not diminish love, will transport us to the furthest shore.*

GOING DEEPER – EXPERIENCING LOSS, DYING AND DEATH AS *MYSTERY*

Accessing this highway Isaiah speaks of can seem terrifying because it involves letting go. Imagine standing at the precipice of a seemingly bottomless pit. Taking this approach involves **descending into the darkness of the unknown**, without the familiar coping mechanisms that have, to some extent, protected you from the harshness of life. Venturing into this pit involves a leap of faith and a sacred surrender. By letting go of what you've been taught to cling to, your hands and heart can finally open enough to receive something new. And that something new is a higher level of consciousness that can transcend the "is what it is" aspect of any significant loss as well as the losses inherent in dying. As you surrender into this mystery you'll experience a greater sense of wholeness and unity with all of creation and the confidence that, in death, your world and your ability to give and receive love will expand exponentially.

Those who cling to the surface of the experience, who judge the quality of their day-to-day existence only in terms of what they've lost or stand to lose, will need to depend more and more on the very coping mechanisms that hold them prisoner, adding emotional pain, mental anguish, and spiritual desolation to their situation. Conversely, those who choose to explore a higher level of consciousness, to surrender into the mystery of their loss, can discover a power greater than themselves that can move them to love in a freedom they've never known before, shifting the focus from self to others, thus alleviating much self-imposed suffering.

This alternate lens is sometimes not the one family or friends will share. It might seem to others as though you're giving up the battle, caving in to circumstance, showing weakness, when in fact taking this view requires great courage and faith. You recognize, clearly, finally, that you are entering into the process of dying (whether it's a relationship, a job, a dream, or actual physical death), and that who you were before will be no more. The person who will later ascend from the darkness of this pit will be a totally new creation, someone you can't yet imagine.

This is what rebirth means. It's terrifying, because it calls us to a stance of *radical surrender.* It feels like a free-fall.

And yet we begin to recognize that the seeds of life, death, and rebirth have been planted deep in the very fiber of our DNA – that, as Jesus said in John 12:24, *"Unless a grain of wheat falls to the ground and dies, it remains just a grain of wheat; but if it dies, it produces much fruit."* These familiar words begin to resonate with profound truth that we were never able to grasp before.

Without this radical letting go it is impossible to carve a space for a new reality. Everything superfluous in life, everything that cloaks us in the "false self," must be stripped away in order for our true selves to be revealed – who we are in God and at the core of our being. When we allow this to happen we begin to enter a higher level of consciousness unavailable to us when we're busy clinging to the 'stuff' of the world. This stripping expands our vision so we can begin to see the bigger picture, can touch into a revelation about the blessed, interconnectedness of all things – a doorway into a whole new level of being. This state of interconnectedness is often referred to as "whole-making." It is what Jesus drew from as he walked the road to Calvary in a loving stance, when he forgave those who betrayed him, what Viktor Frankl was able to tap in order to see goodness and love in the midst of horror.

Read the revelation that Viktor Frankl experienced as he and hundreds of others were being led through the gates of a work camp as revealed in his book, *Man's Search for Meaning*:

A thought transfixed me: for the first time in my life I saw the truth as it is set into song by so many poets, proclaimed as the final wisdom by so many thinkers. The truth--that love is the ultimate and the highest goal to which man can aspire. Then I grasped the meaning of the greatest secret that human poetry and human thought and belief have to impart: The salvation of man is through love and in love. I understood how a man who has nothing left in this world may still know bliss, be it only for a brief moment, in the contemplation of his beloved. In a position of utter desolation, when a man cannot express himself in positive action, when his only achievement may consist in enduring his sufferings in the right way--an honorable way--in such a position man can, through loving contemplation of the image he carries of his beloved, achieve fulfillment. For the first time in my life, I was able to understand the words, "The angels are lost in perpetual contemplation of an infinite glory."

Decades later, under radically different circumstances, another brilliant doctor came to the same conclusion about the power of love. Neurosurgeon Eben Alexander, of Brigham & Women's and Children's Hospitals and Harvard Medical School, suffered from a rare and devastating illness which rendered the neocortex section of his brain nonfunctional. Dr. Alexander fell into a coma and was kept afloat on life support. During this time he had a dramatic 'NDE' or *near death experience* for which there was no neuro-scientific explanation. Dr. Alexander was not a religious man, in fact he was more of a skeptic, and despite this, during his NDE he underwent a transformation of consciousness in which he connected not only to his own spirit or soul, but to what he described as "all that is." He wrote a book about this titled, *Proof of Heaven,* in which he speaks of the revelation he experienced and the clear message he took away from his encounter with God:

You are loved and cherished.
   You have nothing to fear.
   There is nothing you can do wrong.
   If I had to boil it down further, to just one sentence, it would run this way:
   You are loved.
   And if I had to boil it down further, to just one word, it would (of course) be, simply: *Love.*

Love is, without a doubt, the basis of everything. Not some abstract, hard-to-fathom kind of love but the day-to-day kind that everyone knows – the kind of love we feel when we look at our spouse and our children, or even our animals. In its purest and most powerful form, this love is not jealous or selfish, but *unconditional.* This is the reality of realities, the incomprehensibly glorious truth of truths that lives and breathes at the core of everything that exists or that ever will exist, and no remotely accurate understanding of who and what we are can be achieved by anyone who does not know it, and embody it in all of their actions.

First, a Jewish psychiatrist and, decades later, an American agnostic neurosurgeon arrived at the same conclusion - that the essence of life was to love. Frankl and Alexander are, of course, not the only ones who've experienced this revelation. Almost a hundred years earlier, in the late 19th century, Carmelite sister Therese of Lisieux "The Little Flower" embodied the same ideal.

This unpretentious, high-spirited young French woman joined the convent at age 15. Her life up to that point had not been easy – her mother died when Therese was four, leaving her in the care of her beloved sister Pauline. Five years later Pauline joined the Carmelite order. In the months that followed, Therese suffered from a fever so severe that her family didn't expect her to live. After she pulled through, two more of her sisters left for the convent as well. As a teenager Therese struggled with tremendous self-doubt. She begged to join the convent, and when she was finally allowed her romanticized notions of convent life were shattered – she was met with cold rudeness by some within her community. While there her father suffered a mental breakdown and was institutionalized. Therese sustained herself through mental prayer and seeking "sweetness" in suffering. In 1896 she was afflicted with tuberculosis. Her pain was unrelenting – so much so that she claimed in her autobiography *The Story of a Soul*, that had it not been for her faith she might have taken her own life: "What a grace it is to have faith! If I had no faith, I would have inflicted death on myself without hesitating a moment."

Despite her suffering, her legacy was this – that throughout her short life (she died at age 24) she sought to love in all encounters – even in dealing with the most difficult people and trying circumstances. The essence of her book, which has been translated into over 60 languages and in print for more than century, can be encapsulated as follows:

Pain, Pleasure: I embrace them both the same way. With love. Love contains within itself every possible vocation. Love is everything. Love embraces all time and all space. Love is eternal. So in the height of joy, I cry out in a frenzy: "O Jesus, beloved! My vocation, at last I have found it. My vocation is to love."

The Divine Paradox
Isn't it curious that it was through suffering that Victor Frankel, Eben Alexander, and Therese, the Little Flower, all had powerful revelations about love? It made me wonder what love and suffering have in common. It's a compelling question.

At first, love and suffering seem incongruent. Unless your heart's been broken, love is bliss, or, if not bliss, at least mutually satisfying – isn't that how we look at it? This may be true at the beginning stages of romantic love. But ask anyone who's been married for more than a few years and the answer may be very different.

In our dualistic minds we tend to think of suffering as 'bad' and loving as 'good.' Love is desirable, suffering is something to avoid. But, digging deeper reveals that love and suffering have more than a little in common. Both involve mystery. Both require an emptying of or dying to self. When we suffer, we're forced to face our vulnerabilities, losses, and mortality. *And we do the same in love* – we become vulnerable to the other, we sacrifice for the other, we die to our own desires and needs in deference to the other. If we aren't willing to suffer, we're not willing to love – as Simon and Garfunkel expressed in their iconic song *I am a Rock:*

I am shielded in my armor,
Hiding in my room, safe within my womb.
I touch no one and no one touches me.
I am a rock,
I am an island.
And a rock feels no pain;
And an island never cries.

To be open to love is to consent to suffering. As parents gaze at their new-born child they're often blown away by this realization – how exposed they are to vulnerability, how frightened they are at the potential loss of this child, how their own mortality might affect their responsibilities to this new life. This daunting realization sometimes causes parents or lovers to withdraw in an unconscious move toward self-preservation. And if they do, they can never love.

Frankl, Alexander, and Therese all faced circumstances in which they were extremely vulnerable, in which they were forced to relinquish all the things that defined them, stripping them of their identity and sense of security, leaving them completely ungrounded. At the same time they opened themselves to a new type of freedom – freedom from the Prison of Self, from all the striving, from the attachments of life, of culture, of expectations, of ego, of the exhausting need to control. *The underpinning of that radical freedom is love.*

Is it realistic to expect "regular people" to aspire to this kind of loving in the face of great suffering? Most would agree that it's difficult even in the best of times, impossible when faced with the challenges and anxieties inherent in the dying process.

Perhaps a deeper understanding of the nature of the God within can help us take this radical step toward loving out of our suffering. In the next chapter we'll explore the nature of God and the tough questions about the role God plays in the unfolding of life.

CHAPTER 13

Who is This God Within?

AS HUMAN BEINGS, consciously or unconsciously, we thirst to know the God that dwells within us. Not to know *about* God, but to *know* God, to have a personal encounter with God. And, to believe that as much as we thirst for God – God thirsts for us. What sustained Saint Teresa of Calcutta in her ministry serving the poorest of the poor was a revelation she received on the train to Darjeeling in 1946. In a transformative moment she was overwhelmed by God's presence, and received a clear message about the nature of God:

> "He longs for you. He thirsts for you...My children, once you have experienced the thirst, the love of Jesus for you, you will never need, you will never thirst for these things which can only lead you away from Jesus, the true and living Fountain. Only the thirst of Jesus, feeling it, hearing it, answering it with all your heart will keep your love...alive. The closer you come to Jesus the better you will know His thirst."

Who is this God that thirsts for us? And how do we experience this God for whom we thirst?

Early on in my ministry, not long after my experience with Chester (the old man who opened my eyes to how little I knew about standing with the sick and dying) I had another intense encounter with a parishioner. Valerie's young son had drowned in a pond behind her house. I was called to try to help the family come to terms with the unimaginable. I rang the bell, and was ushered into the living room. Friends and family were seated around Valerie, trying to console her. When she saw me she rose from the couch. I stepped forward to offer an embrace. Instead she came at me, pummeled me with her fists, pounded my chest. I had to raise my arms to protect my face. "I *hate* God!" she yelled. "I *hate* him!"

Trying to reconcile a tragic event with the idea of an all-powerful and all-loving God is difficult. For centuries philosophers and theologians have struggled with it. The untold suffering in the world, and the losses we all have to deal with give us cause to pause. Why would a loving God, a God who asks us to call him Father, Abba – *Daddy* – allow us to suffer as we do? Doesn't this seem to fly in the face of scripture? In Matthew 7:9-11 Jesus said,

> *"Which one of you would hand his son a stone when he asks for a loaf of bread, or a snake when he asks for a fish? If you then, who are wicked, know how to give good gifts to your children, how much more will your heavenly father give good things to those who ask him?"*

Surely Valerie felt as though she'd been given worse than a stone or a snake. She felt that God had snatched her son from her. And she had no use for such a God.

OUR LIVES AS PASCHAL MYSTERY

Without a doubt, the world we live in is broken. You don't need to look far to see suffering. In my ministry I've discovered that even the people who seem to have it all together bear their share of private pain and silent anguish. Everyone, without exception, carries a story of loss.

As a priest, I'm often teased about having a cushy job – "Must be nice to only work on Sundays." Nothing could be further from the truth. In a typical week in my parish, babies are baptized, a wedding consecrated, a relationship comes undone, an annulment is granted, the sick anointed, and the dead honored and prepared for burial. The Paschal Mystery plays out, again and again – and I continually witness the cycle of birth, dying, and rising that is at the heart of Christian teaching. Out of darkness comes light. Out of death, life. This Paschal Mystery is observed every year during Holy Week and unfolds over and over again in the messiness of our lives, but we often don't have the eyes to see it. Each time it brings me back to the parallels between love and suffering. Both spring from the same root, from the natural cycle of life.

Another manifestation of the inherent connection between joy and suffering strikes me whenever I take in something of great beauty – a spectacular sunset, the waves crashing against the shore, birdsong in the morning, the sun dancing on the water. The joy that I feel always has a bittersweet edge of loss, an undercurrent of longing, of something somehow unfulfilled, something deeper than what meets the eye. The beauty of God's creation embodies this mysterious synergy of the cycle of life and death. It also suggests that humanity is just one part of a much bigger reality – that we, all the universe, and whatever lies beyond it are connected, and that all participate in the great dance of dying and rising that is the Paschal Mystery.

We witness this day in and day out. Yet, when faced with our own losses, with the decay and decline of what we treasure, we look to God to make us the exception, and beg him to let us sit out our turn in the dance. I thought of this one recent Sunday. The reading was from Matthew 6:25-34 where Jesus tells us not to worry or be anxious because, after all, doesn't God care for the flowers of the field and the birds? How much more, he asks, does God love us, his daughters and sons? Yet, I think, don't the flowers droop and fade? Doesn't the sparrow die? We know this, yet our pleas to God are rooted much more in hope for the continuation of what we know than in faith and confidence in the God of a bigger, richer reality.

SHRINKING GOD TO OUR SIZE

There's a powerful parallel between adults standing before the mystery of who God is (or what heaven is like) and an unborn child in the womb. Both have become comfortable with the world as they know it. Neither wants to leave the familiarity and security of that place. For the unborn child there are occasional hints of something beyond the warm, wet, well-insulated realm in which he floats – a muffled sound, gentle pressure. But life outside the womb is *so* much greater than the fetal imagination can grasp. Likewise, we sometimes sense a greater reality than the tangible world before us – when we stand in the beauty of nature, witness the birth of a child, hear words of love or a strain of music that touches us at our core – at the fringes of our consciousness we might sense the existence of a powerful, all-loving presence. Instead of reaching toward this in faith we tend to restrict our understanding of God to the tiny perimeters of our own imagination and experience.

> In J.B. Phillips' classic *Your God is Too Small: A Guide for Believers and Skeptics Alike,* he says: "Many men and women today are living, often with inner dissatisfaction, without any faith in God at all. This is not because they are particularly wicked or selfish, or, as the old-fashioned would say, "godless" but because they have not found with their adult minds a God big enough to "account for" life, big enough to "fit in with" the new scientific age, big enough to command their highest admiration and respect, and consequently their willing cooperation."

We constrain our vision of God to our own limited perspective, and fight against accepting a reality rooted in a much broader mystery. We have a tendency to make God into a puppeteer or an absentee landlord, a policeman or a fairy godmother who either dishes out blessings and punishments or ignores us altogether. Perhaps the reality is something we simply don't have the capacity to fathom. Because of the narrow scope of our view, we project onto God our own inadequate ability to love. We typically pick and choose who we'll love, or offer love only when certain conditions are met. Sometimes we hurt those we profess to love, or when someone we love hurts us we lash out or withdraw from them. So, on some level, we assume that God does the same, especially when we look honestly at our own faults and un-loveable-ness. Why should we receive more than we can deliver? In the human view, it seems improbable, but Scripture tells us differently – that, thankfully, God's ways are not ours.

WHAT DO WE KNOW ABOUT THE NATURE OF GOD?

Through the years I've sat with many parents who struggled with their children's problems – drugs, alcohol, addictions of all kinds, serious mental illness from which they just couldn't recover. One mother came to me after her son had died - a middle-aged man who was unable to beat his alcohol addiction. He'd ended up homeless, and his mother had often had to respond to him with tough love. In the end, he wandered onto a highway, was hit by a truck, and killed. She came to my office and spoke of her boy, tears in her eyes, reflecting on not only his struggles, but his childhood, before things went awry. "Father," she said, looking at me with riveting intensity, "Through it all I just loved him so."

I was awed by this, struck by the significance of her words, and the depth and purity of her unconditional love and mercy for him. "Mary Fran," I said to her, "You just revealed to me the very face of God."

This was a scenario I'd witnessed many times, the circumstances and faces changing, but the overwhelming love of a parent for a child, even a very broken child, surpassed all else.

If, in our human weakness, this kind of parental love is possible, how much more so is God's love for us? We are, after all, referred to as "children of God."

In 1John 4:7-8 we hear: *Beloved, let us love one another, because love is of God; everyone who loves is begotten by God and knows God. Whoever is without love does not know God, for God is love.*

And this is far from the only Scriptural reference about the loving nature of God. In fact, there are far too many passages to include here.

But, if you're still skeptical – if you feel you haven't experienced this love first hand, or perhaps it seems a little too easy to simply claim that God is a loving God, especially when this flies in the face of your life experience, keep this in mind: Barbara has reminded me that authors always talk about the power of "showing" rather than "telling." It's one thing to tell the reader that God is love, it's another to show this clearly. The best way to do this is to look at not only what Jesus said, but what he *did*.

Jesus: God's Love Personified

I'm continually struck by Jesus' immense compassion for those who were hurting, especially the marginalized, the outcast, the alienated. This compassion led to action, which put him at odds with the established authority of his time. He demonstrated this compassion by his willingness to dialogue in a non-violent way with those who were determined to undermine him. Even as the pressure from his opponents intensified, he remained in a loving stance toward them. He sought to turn the norm of the day - "an eye for an eye and a tooth for tooth" - upside down, replacing it with the image of "turning the other cheek."

At the Last Supper, Jesus washed the feet of his disciples, performing a menial task with great love, a symbolic act rooted in forgiveness, knowing they would betray, deny, and abandon him. Clearly, Jesus represents the pinnacle of compassionate love in the face of adversity. He was a model of how to love unconditionally, whatever the circumstance. What empowered him to do this was the fact that he knew he was loved in the same way by his God. Pope Francis, in His Apostolic Letter: Misericordia et misera (November 20, 2016), captured this understanding:

"Forgiveness is the most visible sign of the Father's love, which Jesus sought to reveal by his entire life. Every page of the Gospel is marked by this imperative of a love that loves to the point of forgiveness. Even at the last moment of his earthly life, as he was being nailed to the cross, Jesus spoke words of forgiveness: "Father, forgive them; for they know not what they do." (Lk 23:34) Nothing of what a repentant sinner places before God's mercy can be excluded from the embrace of his forgiveness. For this reason, none of us has the right to make forgiveness conditional. Mercy is always a gratuitous act of our heavenly Father, an unconditional and unmerited act of love. Consequently, we cannot risk opposing the full freedom of the love with which God enters into the life of every person. Mercy is this concrete action of love that, by forgiving, transforms and changes our lives. In this way, the divine mystery of mercy is made manifest. God is merciful (cf. Ex 34:6); his mercy lasts forever (cf. Ps 136). From generation to generation, it embraces all those who trust in him and it changes them, by bestowing a share in his very life."

Likewise, Saint Pope John Paul II said, "Mercy is love's second name."

JESUS' DIRECTIVE TO LOVE - A MIRROR OF GOD'S LOVE AND MERCY FOR US

It's equally compelling to look at how Jesus instructs *us* to love, because if, in our human weakness, we're expected to love this way, *how much greater must God's love be for us?* Jesus certainly wouldn't hold us to a higher standard than God's.

What Jesus taught about the way to love goes far beyond what we see as fair or adequate. His directive to love is radical, expansive, and all-inclusive, constantly pushing and pulling us across the boundaries we erect between ourselves and others. In Luke 6:27 Jesus proclaims,

"But to you who hear I say, love your enemies, do good to those who hate you, bless those who curse you, pray for those who mistreat you. To the

person who strikes you on one cheek, offer the other one as well, and from the person who takes your cloak, do not withhold your tunic. Give to everyone who asks of you, and from the one who takes what is yours, do not demand it back. Do to others as you would have them do to you. For if you love those who love you, what credit is that to you? Even sinners love those who love them. And if you do good to those who do good to you, what credit is that to you? Even sinners do the same. If you lend money to those from whom you expect repayment, what credit is that to you? Even sinners lend to sinners and get back the same amount. But rather, love your enemies and do good to them, and lend expecting nothing back; then your reward will be great and you will be children of the Most High, for he himself is kind to the ungrateful and the wicked. Be merciful, just as your Father is merciful."

Jesus also says, in Matthew 18:21-22 that we must forgive endlessly. Peter asks him:

"Lord, if my brother sins against me how often must I forgive him? As many as seven times?" Jesus answered, "I say to you not seven times, but seventy seven times."

In other words, he is telling us, figuratively, that we must forgive as often as we are wronged.

In his book, *Mercy: The Essence of the Gospel and the Key to Christian Life*, Cardinal Walter Kasper writes: "It is clear: love of one's enemy is perhaps the most humanly difficult demand of Jesus yet it is, at the same time, one of the most central Christian commandments. It is rooted in the innermost essence of the Christian mystery and, therefore, represents the specific character of Christian behavior."

Cardinal Kasper is right – and, sadly, we generally dismiss this funda-mental teaching at the heart of Gospel because it seems impossible to live out by broken people in a broken world. So, we minimize the mes-sage, think of it as nothing more than an idealistic platitude meant to inspire us. The tragedy in this is that by dismissing this teaching, *we also dismiss the fact that this is the way God relates to us!*

THE EMPOWERMENT OF KNOWING GOD'S LOVE

As we begin to recognize that God loves us, that God thirsts for us, and that we are one with love itself, everything changes. In the Gospel of John he writes: *Those who love know God.* He doesn't say, "Those who know God, love." Our willingness to love is prerequisite to the knowing. The way to really know God is to follow Jesus' directive – to love, radically. And love is an action, a verb – not a feeling. It is conscious, intentional, difficult. It always requires an emptying of self.

This outward movement of reaching out in love has a reciprocal inner movement. As we relate, in love, to those around us, we journey deeper toward the God within. Pope Francis noted this dynamic: "Whenever we encounter another person in love, we learn something new about God." As we love, our hearts are opened in a greater way to the presence and action of God in our lives. As we love we live out the Christian paradox - in giving, we receive. In dying to self, we live in greater wholeness and freedom. As our willingness to love expands, so does our image of God. Our thirst is finally satiated by the object of our hidden longing. This, in turn, empowers us to continue to love in deeper ways.

The question is: Is it possible to begin to expand our ability to love in this way when our losses, our illness, and our grief feel all-encompassing?

CHAPTER 14

The Fertile Patch – God's Love is at Work in Everyone

I ALWAYS SAY that in every heart there's a field where the seeds of unconditional love have been sown and cultivated. It's from this secret garden that God's power germinates and grows, creating a push and pull toward wholeness that continually seeks to move us toward an ever-expansive love for others. Our true self is rooted in this field, in perfect union with God and with all that is.

Unfortunately, more often than not, we fail to recognize the rich soil of this field because it's largely hidden under rocks, hard packed soil, and bramble. In Matthew, chapter 13, Jesus refers to this in the "Parable of the Sower":

> A sower went out to sow. And as he sowed, some seed fell on the path, and birds came and ate it up. Some fell on rocky ground, where it had little soil. It sprang up at once because the soil was not deep and when the sun rose it was scorched, and it withered for lack of roots. Some seed fell among thorns, and the thorns grew up and choked it. But some seed fell on rich soil, and produced fruit, a hundred or sixty or thirtyfold. Whoever has ears ought to hear.

The rich soil represents our oneness with and the working of God in our lives. The rocks are the unhealed emotional wounds we've received from others, from ourselves, or from life. Perhaps someone has belittled, shamed, or disregarded us. We may have been betrayed or rejected by a loved one, disappointed by life, emotionally, physically, or sexually abused. In addition, we forget that when we hurt others we also are hurting ourselves - the hurt given is also measured back to us. These become the hidden wounds of our hearts. As we rationalize why we're justified in hurting someone else, these self-inflicted hidden hurts ravage us like a silent cancer.

When the field of our heart is littered with this kind of rubble, we become stuck. Instead of moving forward in freedom we focus on the past, hobbling over the stones of our hurts. When we try to side-step this rocky ground we end up retreading the same worn patch of soil. Large sections of the field become hard-packed and impermeable, making it difficult for us to receive and give love.

Think of the bramble and thorns as the negative defensive behaviors we engage in to protect ourselves from further hurts heaped upon any unhealed emotional wounds. I explain it this way... Imagine you have an open wound on your hand. What do you do if someone reaches out to you? You pull your hand back. If they persist, you'll push them away with negative or aggressive behaviors, or completely retreat. We do this to protect ourselves, and in the process, hurt others. We suffer injury upon injury, and our fear of being hurt again causes even greater worry and pain. Consciously or unconsciously we transmit our suffering to others by pushing them away or lashing out at them. Wracked with guilt or shame, we might turn the pain inward, and begin imaging ourselves in negative terms: I'm a loser, a failure, a push-over. As we identify more and more with these self-destructive labels, they begin to color our interactions. Unintentionally, our behavior aligns with our self-image, perpetuating the negative cycle. When those around us fail to recognize the pain that drives the behavior, they either steer clear or react in adverse ways.

We're all, in varying degrees, handicapped by the rubble that litters the inner fields of our hearts. Combined with the challenges of an illness it can begin to feel overwhelming. At the same time, this cumulative pain can serve a positive purpose. The suffering we experience *can* be transformative, if we have the eyes to see.

THE REDEMPTIVE POWER OF SUFFERING

All the great spiritual traditions talk about the redemptive, transformative power of suffering. As the late American preacher E.H. Chapin said, "Out of suffering have emerged the strongest souls; the most massive characters are seared with scars." Yet, what sane person would invite suffering, even as a vehicle for healing and transformation? An extremist perhaps, a martyr, or a masochist. What's so difficult is that while we all would gladly avoid suffering, (even Jesus, in the Garden of Gethsemane, prayed for the cup to pass him by) it's an inevitable part of life.

At first glance suffering seems pointless. By its very nature, suffering threatens the ego self – our survival, self-interest, and/or self-definition. We go to great extremes to prevent or alleviate it. Clearly, if we're operating out of the ego self, suffering will be seen as worthless, and to be avoided at all cost. So, what are the mystics talking about? Where exactly is the value in suffering? And how can it propel us to love?

COMPASSION

If we look at the word 'compassion', breaking it into its roots, it means, literally, "to suffer with." If we haven't personally fallen under the weight of sadness, disappointment, struggle, failure, or sickness, it's hard to genuinely put ourselves in another's shoes. We can sympathize – feeling and expressing sorrow and regret about the situation others find themselves in. Beyond sympathy is empathy, where we can feel not only sorrow, but can really listen to, understand, and commiserate with the other. When we sympathize there's a level of objectivity and psychic distance between us and the person suffering. But the next level - true compassion (rooted in empathy) - can only come after we've embraced our own failings and acknowledged the darkness of our shadow-selves that we'd prefer to hide. By accepting our powerlessness, we can begin to embrace compassion - the depth and breadth of it commensurate with our suffering. We start to see others without judging them; we become less vulnerable to any hurt or rejection at their hands *because we understand their weakness and their sin as we do our own.* We're able to comprehend, first-hand, the pain that drives their behavior. Compassion becomes part of our fiber, radically freeing us to cultivate the sacrificial love we were destined to partake in and share, a love born of suffering.

"Through compassion it is possible to recognize that the craving for love that people feel resides also in our own hearts, that the cruelty the world knows all too well is also rooted in our own impulses. Through compassion we also sense our hope for forgiveness in our friends' eyes and our hatred in their bitter mouths. When they kill, we know that we could have done it; when they give life, we know that we can do the same. For a compassionate person nothing human is alien: no joy and no sorrow, no way of living and no way of dying."

— HENRI J.M. NOUWEN, *THE WOUNDED HEALER*

Similarly, Fr. Richard Rohr refers to our suffering as potentially "sacred wounds."

He says, "If we cannot find a way to make our wounds into sacred wounds, we invariably become negative or bitter—because we will be wounded. That is a given. All suffering is potentially redemptive, all wounds are potentially sacred wounds. It depends on what you do with them. Can you find God in them or not? If there isn't some way to find some deeper meaning to our suffering, to find that God is somehow in it, and can even use it for good, we will normally close up and close down, and the second half of our lives will, quite frankly, be small and silly."

The real hope in all of this lies in the Paschal Mystery – out of darkness, light; out of death, life. The fertile soil inside us where God dwells is constantly drawing us toward compassion and love regardless of whether we're aware of it or not. Despite the number of wounds we've received, despite the rocks and bramble that conceal the richness of this sacred field, there's always a thrust toward greater wholeness and unconditional love. The work of expanding the fertile patch into an entire field is what Victor Frankl talked about. We all have a fertile patch inside, regardless of our struggles and sin. It may be difficult to see, challenging to recognize, littered as it may be with the rocks, bramble, and hard-packed soil of life. God is working, whether you're aware of it or not. Pope Francis talks about this as well:

> "I have a dogmatic certainty: God is in every person's life. God is in everyone's life. Even if the life of a person has been a disaster, even if it is destroyed by vices, drugs, or anything else -- God is in this person's life. You can, you must try to seek God in every human life. Although the life of a person is a land full of thorns and weeds, there is always a space in which the good seed can grow. You have to trust God."

Without a doubt, becoming aware of the fertile patch within is the first step toward expanding it into a bountiful field.

Peter's Story

Rob, a parishioner, stopped by the Parish Center one day to see me. His brother Peter had died and Rob was trying to plan a simple funeral. "He wasn't a practicing Catholic," Rob explained. "In fact, he...well, he wasn't a very nice person." Rob teared up. "He's probably going straight to hell. His life was a mess. Left a trail of pain behind him. So I understand if you can't do the funeral."

I brought Rob into my office and we sat down. "Tell me about your brother," I said.

Rob sighed deeply. "Peter was difficult from start to finish. He was always oppositional, in constant trouble in school. Got messed up with drugs, alcohol. One run-in after another with the police. He dragged my family into all of it. Bailing him out, getting him into rehab, tough love – all of it for nothing." Rob shook his head. "My brother never thought of anyone but himself," he said. "Broke my parents' hearts."

"Rob," I said. "This is a story I've heard more times than I can count. Peter just couldn't get out of his own way."

"Do you think he'll go to hell? " Rob asked.

"None of us earns our way into heaven," I said. I grabbed my pad and drew a large rectangle. Then I added a small circle on the inside edge of the rectangle. I explained to Rob about the parable of the sower, and then asked him to try to see his brother's struggles in a different way – as stones and bramble. Rob was skeptical until I pushed him to try and find some shred of evidence that pointed to the fertile patch – some small act of love and compassion indicating that God was working in his brother's life.

"Well," Rob said, "It isn't much, but…"

"Doesn't need to be much," I prompted.

He went on to tell me about driving his brother to the hospital for cancer treatment. They'd stopped at a traffic light at a busy intersection where homeless people stood and begged. Peter rolled down the window and waved. The homeless man flashed a toothless grin. "Peter!" he called.

"You know him? " Rob had asked.

"He's got nothing," Peter replied. "So I take him for breakfast sometimes."

I raised my eyebrows. "Really? And you think he's going to hell? When was the last time any of us took a homeless man to breakfast?"

Rob shook his head. "Yeah, but…"

"The fertile patch," I said.

"There was another thing," Rob said. "We were in the hospital. I was pushing Peter in the wheelchair and a nurse walked by. Peter started flirting with her - teasing, smiling." Rob nodded, remembering. 'Jeez,

Pete,' I told him, 'even now you're chasing women. Leave her alone!'"
"My brother said, 'Rob, did you see her?' Of course I saw her. But Peter
said, 'Did you *really* see her? The pock marks on her face?'"

Rob's eyes welled. "I hadn't noticed. But Peter persisted. He said, 'I
don't want her feeling bad about herself. So I try and make her smile a
little. Nothin' wrong with that.'"

"Wow," I said. "As much as your brother was a broken instrument,
he had compassion. And God was working through him, although he
wasn't aware of it."

Rob shook his head. "But, then, why did he put the family through
such hell? "

"Expectations," I said. "The little people he reached out to didn't
place any expectations on him. So he felt safe. Didn't worry about letting
them down. The fertile patch was there..."

Rob muffled a sob. "I just never saw it."

"Hard to see," I said. "But there, nonetheless."

We went ahead and planned the funeral. A celebration of the hope
that, beyond the grave, Peter's fertile patch would be, with his consent,
fully cleared, cultivated, and harvested.

Most of us likely look at someone like Peter and think, a little smugly,
"Thank God I'm not anything like that. I take care of my family, work
hard..." But even those of us who are wrapped in much tidier packages
have stones and bramble littering God's fertile field that prevent us from
loving as we're called to...

CARMEN

Denise's mother Carmen was widowed at a young age. With six children
to raise on her own Carmen had to run a tight ship. She took in sewing
and laundry in order to put clothes on their backs and food on their
table. There was little time for Carmen to give Denise and her siblings
the kind of warm attention they craved. Carmen smiled little, worked
long hours, and demanded much from all of the children. It was the
only way to keep the household running.

Denise continually looked for her mother's approval, but seldom received it. In fact, it was quite the opposite. Carmen was critical and punitive, trying to "toughen her up" in order to face whatever life might dish out.

Denise grew up, married, had children of her own. She lived next door to Carmen, and for more than 50 years did the shopping, cared for the lawn and yard, and in later years, the cleaning and laundry for her mother. And yet it was never good enough. The only way Carmen seemed to show her love was through food and by showering her grandchildren with affection. She'd make homemade macaroni, ravioli, eggplant and veal parmesan, gathering the family around her every Sunday. Cannolis for the little ones, or Italian pizzelles. Across the decades, Denise often felt that she'd like to host sometimes, to feel the center of her own home. But Carmen wouldn't hear of it.

By the time Carmen died, Denise had had enough. She had come to resent the old woman, and felt saddled by the weight of obligation in the care she provided. After the funeral Denise came to see me. "I'm an awful person, Father," she cried. "The shameful truth is that I'm relieved she's dead. Most days I just couldn't stand her!"

"Sit down Denise," I said. "I want to show you something." I drew my diagram of the fertile patch. Explained that her mother had a fertile patch – evidence of that was how hard she'd worked to support the family, and the way she lavished her cooking on all of them until she just couldn't stand at the stove any more. She was powered by God's love to somehow get them through.

"Well, all I ever really wanted was a kind word. To be able to laugh together. Maybe a hug." Denise sniffled. "I feel like such an ass," she said. "I'm 67 years old, crying for my mother's attention. She was mean-spirited and cheap in that way."

"I'd feel like you do," I replied. "But she was orphaned as a girl and then widowed and left to care for a slew of you kids. Life played hardball with her early on." I drew some small circles and scribbles. "The rocks and bramble of life's hurts – that's what prevented her from being vulnerable with you. And she just didn't know how to clear the field. It wasn't you, Denise. She was wounded and she couldn't transform it. So she transmitted it, unconsciously."

This opened a floodgate. I reached over and touched Denise's arm, "So, don't be so hard on yourself. Those tears connect you to your mother in compassion. You both, in some ways, shared the same wounds. But now we can begin to remove the rocks and bramble she left in your field. Let's get to work!"

I counseled Denise on how to approach forgiveness and healing, encouraged her to begin "doing little things with great love," and asked her to fast from all negativity. Most importantly, we talked about generational wounds and the importance of transforming these, rather than transmitting them to her own children. (More on all of this in subsequent chapters.)

EMPTY, FILL, AND SPILL

Clearly, one of the bounties of God's fertile field is compassion. Despite the amount of rocks and bramble we carry, this compassion draws us into oneness with everyone, not only by the respect for and appreciation of shared suffering, but by the recognition that within everyone there is this same fertile patch where God and the true self dwell. This new awareness of the incarnation allows us to begin to reach out in mercy, even to those with whom we struggle. This is what Jesus granted Bartimeaus when he asked to be cured of his blindness, when he cried out, "Lord, I want to see." Once we suffer, we can become compassionate, our eyes opened, and we become freer to love – *and this is evidence of God's healing power within us.*

In endeavoring to transform our suffering into "sacred wounds" we realize the possibilities for making closure, bringing peace, offering hope, giving witness to God's light in the dark times, and planting the powerful seeds of unconditional love – this, the most powerful legacy we can leave behind. In essence, our suffering empties us, casting aside the ego, creating a space for God's love to blossom. When we allow this to happen we become vessels for God's unconditional love. As we grow more and more open to this love, it fills us to overflowing, spilling onto everyone and everything we touch. This is the purest of all love, as it flows through us directly from God, transcending the false self, seeking nothing in return. *Empty, fill, and spill* – this can become the dynamic that transforms dying and death into gift for everyone touched by it. The concept of 'empty, fill, and spill' is powerfully reflected in the words of St. Paul:

> *But we hold this treasure in earthen vessels, that the surpassing power may be of God and not from us. We are afflicted in every way, but not constrained; perplexed, but not driven to despair; persecuted, but not abandoned; struck down, but not destroyed; always carrying about in the body the dying of Jesus, so that the life of Jesus may also be manifested in our body. Therefore, we are not discouraged; rather, although our outer self is wasting away, our inner self is being renewed day by day. For this momentary light affliction is producing for us an eternal weight of glory beyond all comparison, as we look not to what is seen but to what is unseen; for what is seen is transitory, but what is unseen is eternal. - 2 Corinthians 4:7-10, 16-18*

When we allow God's love to pour forth from our emptiness, the beneficiaries of this grace become our family, friends, and strangers – even those whose hearts may presently be too bound up to receive it. If not now, then eventually, as their lives unfold, touched by vulnerability, loss, and suffering, the love offered will permeate the walls they've erected – as St. Paul says in 1 Corinthians 13:8, *"Love never fails."* Like a flower pushing through a patch of asphalt, God's spiral of love eventually meets its mark – whether on this side of the grave or beyond.

It's clear that our ability to *empty, fill, and spill* is dependent on the condition of God's field within us. The rocks, brambles, and thorns of our interior field are what block our potential to love in deeper ways.

Recognizing this sacred field within, littered as it may be, is really the beginning of a much deeper, more mature faith - a seasoned faith born of suffering that can set us and those around us free to live and love, unencumbered. What does this seasoned faith look like? And how do we embrace and nurture such a faith?

Mature Faith

"Faith sees brightest in darkness."

-- SOREN KIERKEGAARD

CHAPTER 15

The Seasoning of Faith

IDENTIFYING THE FERTILE patch inside us, no matter what its size, changes everything. The awareness of God's indwelling, the emergence of a deeply known sense that the God of love is working in our lives and caring for us in our brokenness and sin is often a radically new concept. This new understanding that we are and always have been loved and cared for by our God bolsters our spirits with a sense of security and hope that the world cannot offer.

Newfound insight into the nature of God is not, however, the hallmark of a mature and seasoned faith. The disciples of Jesus powerfully illustrate this. In the years they spent with Jesus they observed the way he cared for the poor, the sick, and the dying. They were the recipients of the great patience and compassion Jesus demonstrated as he taught them. And yet, despite being in the presence of Love itself, they wrestled with his message and, more often than not, came up short. Michael Casey, in his book, *Fully Human – Fully Divine*, touches into this:

> "It is evident that Jesus' most intimate followers had made little progress in the inward journey to which he called them. Much resistance remained. Even at a relatively late stage in the Gospel, after so many signs and so much teaching, the disciples manifested a certain imperviousness to the reality of Jesus. Their hearts seem to have become hardened. They were no better than the fickle crowd, or the stiff-necked religious authorities. So much time, so much care, so much affection--and with such a slight result. A quick transit through the earliest Gospels leaves

us no doubt that the twelve were deficient, not only in their attitudes and priorities, but also in their understanding of the things of God."

So, what was it that finally opened the disciples' eyes and hearts, led them toward a seasoned, mature faith? How were they transformed from being simply the beneficiaries of God's love into emissaries for spreading that love to the world?

The answer to that question is at the very core of this book. The difference between naïve and mature faith is that, even when steeped in the knowledge that God is love, *naïve faith is always characterized by a focus on self-interest and control.* Throughout their time with Jesus, the disciples persisted in making him into the Messiah they wanted him to be – the glorious hero who would overthrow the Roman government and restore power to Israel. Jesus became the God of their own making, in line with their own dreams and desires. Their personal agendas prevented them from understanding the heart of the Gospel – that Jesus' message was, and is, primarily about one thing – our responsibility to love in the face of every kind of challenge.

It was only after Jesus' death on a cross, when the disciples retreated - broken, grieving, terrified, full of regret and guilt at their own shortcomings – that they finally surrendered their deeply held notions about God and life and began to see differently. That was when Jesus' words began to resonate in new ways.

It's no coincidence that periods of great suffering often give way to a deeper, more mature understanding of God. This is because suffering shatters our naïve and reasonable faith. We're no different than the disciples. Hold them close to heart as you consider the characteristics of seasoned, mature faith – and assess the condition of your spiritual life at this point in your journey.

As we gauge the depth and maturity of our own faith, let's begin by reflecting on the innate relationship we all have with God, whether we've actively pursued that relationship or largely ignored it. In spite of our "religious past" – what we've done or haven't done - we need to remember that God is greater than our efforts, bigger than our neglect, and that regardless of where we've been – in the Prison of Self or free - we can begin now to cultivate a deeper, more mature relationship with God.

Every person, baptized or not, involved in religious practice or not, has a natural connection to God. This is our birthright – that we are born with God within us. Call it the spirit, the soul, the indwelling, the generative thrust, the fertile patch – it exists at the core of all human beings.

Whether we're conscious of it or not, God is always working in our lives and has been right along. It's God's energy that moves us out of self to approach the mysteries of life in a sense of awe and freedom. Acknowledging this presence allows us to place our own myopic experiences into a bigger story, a more meaningful context. This common spirit we all share, consciously or unconsciously, is what helps us relate to others, form friendships, and experience deep, committed, passionate love. Have you ever wondered what it is that soars in us when we gaze on a sunrise or mountain summit, an ocean vista or red-rock canyon? It's what makes even the most cynical among us pray when the plane we're on hits serious turbulence. It's what rises in the unlikely hero who selflessly reaches out to rescue a stranger. It's what empowered Peter, whom we met in the last chapter, to reach beyond his brokenness to care for others. It's sometimes what we fight against as it tugs at us when we experience love - what we dismiss as sentimentality, naiveté, or wishful thinking.

In the dying process it's this divine energy that moves us from denial to resignation, and then on to a state of acceptance. And, if nurtured, it can eventually carry us toward a life (and death) altering transformation.

THE BRIDGE TO MATURE, SEASONED FAITH

The crumbling of naïve and/or reasonable faith is unnerving, but it's a challenge that should be seen as a gift. It calls us through the doorway into darkness, where the mystery of God is revealed in a greater way. Theologian and psychiatrist Gerald May talks about this in his book *The Dark Night of the Soul*:

> To guide us toward the love that we most desire, we must be taken where we could not and would not go on our own. And lest we sabotage the journey, we must not know where we are going. Deep in the darkness, way beneath our senses, God is instilling "another, better love, and "deeper, more urgent longings" that empower our willingness for all necessary relinquishments along the way." When we cannot chart our own course, we become vulnerable to God's protection, and the darkness becomes a "guiding night," a "night more kindly than the dawn."

Linda's and Bob's stories in Chapter 2 are examples of how their respective "dark nights of the soul" transformed them. It is a process that occurs when we're led into the mystery of suffering or darkness, and emerge on the other side more free, less blind, with a greater capacity to love in any situation. The experience of moving through the paradox of "enlightening darkness" is a *conversion experience*. Before the conversion, we stood in what we thought was light, but we were blind, so, regardless of the light we lived in darkness. During conversion, as we stand in the black of night where we expect to be blind, we regain our sight, perceiving what we couldn't before. Once we truly see we can begin to accept our helplessness and our inability to control our situation by filling our emptiness with a power greater than ourselves. Remember Rocco, whom we met at the very beginning of the book? He is the perfect example of a person who moved from naïve and reasonable faith to a mature faith steeped in suffering – and in great joy.

Ritually, in the Christian tradition, this transformation is represented every year on Holy Saturday, when the lights in the church are extinguished and we stand expectantly in the gloom. The Easter candle is lit from an open fire and carried into the body of the church – light breaking forth in darkness.

WHAT MATURE, SEASONED FAITH LOOKS LIKE

Any sustained ordeal naturally shatters our childish notions of who God is and what life is all about. In a depleted state we're forced to face our vulnerability, losses, and mortality, and through suffering we begin to better understand, firsthand, the suffering of others. This is the place where compassion grows, along with a new awareness of and respect for the oneness we share with all humanity. Most of our lives we've spent trying to distinguish ourselves from others, cultivating our uniqueness. With mature faith comes the understanding that while we remain individuals we're also one in heart and soul with *everyone*, continually learning to live in the creative tension between individuality and ever greater one-ness.

With these unfolding insights, hard-won and bittersweet, we begin to stitch a patchwork of seasoned, mature faith born of lived experience in the face of great mystery. All pat assumptions and neat assertions about the nature of life and God have been put to the test and cast aside. You begin to realize that the ability to control life (and death) is really an illusion. As a result, the person you once were is gone. The old paradigm of your life is no longer relevant. Nothing seems to fit anymore. As Jesus said in Mark 2:21:

No one sews a piece of unshrunken cloth on an old cloak. If he does, its fullness pulls away, the new from the old, and the tear gets worse.

Someone new has been birthed out of this death. You've changed. Become seasoned. A new creation. Therefore the way you look at life and death also changes. Finally you begin to see that your lived experience is at the heart of the Gospel. The scripture takes on new meaning still again:

"Unless a grain of wheat falls to the ground and dies, it remains just a grain of wheat. But if it dies, it produces much fruit." – John 12:24

The Bible is no longer a rule book on how to earn God's love, but a roadmap that validates and sanctifies the challenges of loving, living, and dying. We can begin to embrace the cycle of birth, death, and rising that moves the world and all life within it forward. It is time to accept our role in the beautiful and poignant dance of life, and to do it with a gracious heart.

We don't achieve seasoned, mature faith by crossing some line in the sand. Gradually, through our surrendering, we evolve toward it. As we relinquish our illusion of control we begin to hold questions rather than hang on to answers. The person with seasoned, mature faith finds it much harder to divvy up the world in terms of good or bad, right or wrong, black or white. The perspective through the eyes of mature faith contains a lot of gray areas that are much more "and/but" than they are "this/that". The tapestry of mature faith is embroidered with seeming contradictions that peacefully coexist.

Mature faith is less about adhering to the tenets of doctrine than it is about following Jesus' directive to *love*. In one sense it's so much simpler, and in another, so much more difficult. You begin to realize and accept that you'll fall short a lot, as will those around you, but that this doesn't compromise God's love in the least. It also doesn't have to thwart your ability to love. You fall, once, twice, three times, and get up again. You develop a healthy humility through which you appreciate and tolerate the shortcomings of others. You stop trying to earn God's love and concentrate instead on loving others – and in doing so your recognition and experience of God's presence in your life increases. The focus of seasoned mature faith is an orientation of unconditional love toward others. This outward movement takes the place of self-absorption and control. In the process you begin to *know God*, rather than simply *knowing about* God.

FAITH AND DOUBT

The irony is that mature faith is characterized by a lot less certainty. I think author Anne Lamott hit the nail on the head when she talks about faith and doubt - that the opposite of faith isn't doubt – the opposite of faith is *certainty*. She's right – if we were certain, why would we need faith? Pope Francis has also weighed in on the question of faith. After admitting that he has had doubts "many times" he said,

> "We do not need to be afraid of questions and doubts because they are the beginning of a path of knowledge and going deeper; one who does not ask questions cannot progress either in knowledge or in faith."

In light of this we might want to redefine faith as *the place where doubt and belief coexist*. This tension is always present, which is why faith is never easy. It's why we often talk about a "leap of faith" – the leap referring to our willingness to suspend our disbelief and persist in the face of skepticism. This is affirmed in Hebrews 11:1:

> *Faith is the realization of what is hoped for and evidence of things not seen.*

I love the story in Mark 9:22-23, in which a man approaches Jesus and asks him if he can cure his son, saying:

> *"If you can do anything, have compassion on us and help us." Jesus said to him, "If you can! Everything is possible to the one who has faith." Then the boy's father cried out, "I believe, help my unbelief!"*

The man didn't allow his doubt to prevent him from taking a leap of faith. His exclamation that encompasses the tension between faith and doubt can become our prayer of intention: *I believe, help my unbelief!*

Taking a leap of faith begins with *hope* and *intention,* and is fueled by a desire to *see* differently. To shift the paradigm. It propels us to span the chasm of unknowing and grab hold of faith on the other side, like jumping off a ledge without a safety net. In this regard a terminal illness can be freeing – you no longer need a safety net, as you have little left to lose.

So, why not leap? Why not hope? Why not act as though you had the faith you desire? Suspend your disbelief? Think of it as walking on water. Entering through the narrow gate. Meeting God halfway. The vulnerability and courage involved in opening the channels for God's healing, in turn, empowers us to love in new and deeper ways. It allows us to finally cooperate with the generative thrust of God's love that has been moving us through the tough times of our lives from the very beginning – the only difference being that now we begin to have the eyes to see.

OUR TENDENCY TO FORGET

Sadly, regardless of our experience of God's healing love, forgiveness, and grace, we have a tendency to forget. We can easily slip back into the practicalities and demands of life and allow them to dominate. Our faith can be seasoned, but unless it's nurtured we can backslide into naïve and reasonable faith, or even find ourselves back in the Prison of Self.

This tendency to forget is illustrated over and over again in the scriptures. In the Old Testament, the Lord had protected the Israelites, empowering Moses to lead them out of Egypt into the desert, parting the Red Sea, providing them with manna to eat, and water to drink. Still, as soon as they were faced with another difficulty the Israelites forgot that God had, time and again, proven faithful, and they turned away from him, regressing to a simplistic, naïve faith.

Here is God's observation, from Exodus 32:8-9:

> They have soon turned aside from the way I pointed out to them, making for themselves a molten calf and worshipping it, sacrificing to it and crying out, 'This is your God, O Israel, who brought you out of the land of Egypt!' I see how stiff-necked this people is, continued the Lord to Moses.

Since we're not all that different from the Israelites, how can we ensure that our memories won't fail us? That we won't stray once again from being children of God to children of the culture? That our seasoned faith born of suffering won't be diminished by spiritual amnesia?

In the next chapter we'll look at the dispositions necessary to nurture and deepen our faith, to keep our seasoned, more mature faith alive, whether we're in the throes of a serious illness or providing care and support to someone who is. Best of all, if these dispositions can be incorporated into our day-to-day living during what I call "the green times of life" when things are going well, we'd all be better prepared for the losses that life inevitably presents.

CHAPTER 16

Foundations for Spiritual Growth

LEARNING HOW TO let go of much of what you hold near and dear is incredibly difficult. Even if you recognize the value of surrender and aspire to move in that direction, it's impossible to do without deepening your connection to and reliance on God.

Fortunately, every religion includes spiritual traditions that have proven, over time, to be helpful for people trying to access God. These traditions also help us, as forgetful humans, to remember the myriad ways God has been there for us through the ages. Interestingly, the spiritual practices of all the major religions share certain characteristics that have been fruitful for practitioners across the centuries. A spiritual practice can be defined as *a tool for heightening the awareness of God within everyday living, imbuing the sacred into the ordinary.* But before embarking on these practices there are three **spiritual dispositions** that will serve to not only raise our awareness of God, but to help us continue the process of emptying ourselves of everything that stands in the way of our ability to love unconditionally: *awareness, intention, and consent.*

AWARENESS

First, we have to become *aware* of the need to ground our egos in something greater than ourselves. Suffering is often the harbinger of this, as our coping mechanisms and naïve faith fail us. Or, we might be looking at the world from inside the Prison of Self. Situations that challenge our sense of security, esteem, and survival typically activate legions of negative voices inside. This inner chatter snatches us from the present moment, dominating our minds and creating a climate of radical self-absorption.

It's important to create some psychic distance between ourselves and our feelings - to be able to acknowledge a strong emotion without drowning in it. We need to cultivate the detachment that can set us free from the tyranny of the enflamed emotions that block our ability to recognize God's working in our lives. We become aware of a hunger and thirst for something new, something deeply and universally relevant. This begins to pulsate within us, opening the doorway to a more mature and seasoned faith.

INTENTION

This awareness leads us to *intention.* With the help of a spiritual guide we can consider how to proceed, and then make a daily commitment to take some kind of action. A vital and active faith community, a priest, minister, rabbi, imam, Buddhist monk, or spiritual director can sustain you in this quest. A trusted friend or prayer partner can gently help keep your intention before you when life is challenging.

In the absence of these, this book can offer direction and encouragement. Intention must be established in faith – *choosing to believe we will act even as we doubt that we can.* We renew our intention daily, maybe hourly.

CONSENT

The other essential ingredient in any spiritual practice is *consent.* Consent to an openness to the working of God within, consent to trust in rather than judge, manipulate, or control the process. We have to recognize that the spiritual practices we're about to discuss are not rooted in willpower, or in self-discipline, but in surrender and hope. They are completely dependent on our willingness to consent to and have faith in *God's* strength, *God's* love, *God's* grace. To keep us mindful of this we need to continually acknowledge and consent to the power and presence of God within ourselves and in the situation we face.

THE FOUR "S" PRACTICES: SURRENDER, SOLITUDE, SILENCE, SIMPLIFICATION

Once you've nurtured awareness, intention, and consent, it's time to commit to a consistent spiritual practice.

It's important to consider the word 'practice'. It implies that whatever we engage in spiritually isn't intended to be perfect. That's why it requires conscious repetition, with what the Buddhists call "beginners' mind," leaving preconceived notions and expectations at the door, being open to possibilities we cannot yet imagine. Spiritual practice is unlike most of the goal-driven endeavors we've undertaken in our lives. We don't engage in spiritual practice to master it, or to use it as a means to an end. We don't try to surpass others in our practice or to tally points for heaven. We practice for one reason only – to empty ourselves *of* ourselves, to clear away the rubble that blocks our ability to recognize the God of Love working in the reality of our situation. Consenting to this Presence, we begin to let go of anything that hinders it.

There are many spiritual practices – volumes of books have been devoted to them, and people often spend their entire lives deepening these practices. In the Christian tradition, there's Meditation or Centering Prayer, Lectio Divina, the Ignatian Examen, Eucharistic Adoration, the recitation of the Rosary, the Divine Mercy Chaplet, to name just a few. At the heart of all of these is what I call the 4 "S" steps. If you haven't engaged in any consistent practice during the "green times," it can be difficult to begin with the classic practices during the challenges of a serious loss, illness, or impending death. The four "S" steps can be thought of as the foundational gateways to spiritual practice, and I've found that they're simple and effective in affording people access to a much deeper awareness of God in their lives.

The counter-intuitive aspect of these 4 "S" practices is that they're designed, not to fill you, but to *empty* you. To create an opening by clearing away the self-absorption, anxiety, negative and obsessive thoughts that block an awareness of the working of God in your life. Given the pervasiveness of the stones, bramble and weeds, this tilling of the spiritual field isn't an overnight process – it's a daily undertaking, a little like housekeeping. Something you continually pick at, knowing the job is never really done. Some days you might not move a single stone or manage to cut back any of the thorns. But that doesn't matter – your awareness, intention, and consent will suffice. It's a case in which the means are more important than the end – because there is no end. It's all about the process. Not something we finally accomplish or attain. It's about letting go rather than grabbing hold. Simply consenting to the four S practices helps us to remember who we are in God, and diminishes our oppressive attachment to our ego selves. In this way, a spiritual practice is not only counter-intuitive – it's counter-cultural, contrary to most of our worldly pursuits. Your practice becomes *a way of being* that subtly changes the lens through which you view your world.

SURRENDER

First we need to overcome the negative connotation of the word "surrender." During a serious, chronic, or terminal illness we're constantly told to keep fighting – in other words, never give up or give in because surrender is synonymous with losing, waving the white flag in defeat.

As a spiritual practice, surrender is viewed very differently. In place of an antagonistic, offensive stance, surrender can be embraced as a peaceful way to hand all things over to God in order to experience a greater sense of balance and peace.

In an address to the Harvard Medical School, Philip Simmons, PhD, who suffered and later died of ALS (Lou Gehrig's disease), spoke of this from personal experience:

"At one time or another, each of us confronts an experience so powerful, bewildering, joyous, or terrifying that all our efforts to see it as a problem are futile. Each of us reaches the end of reason's rope. And, when we do, we can either grip harder and get nowhere or we can let go and fall. For what does mystery ask of us? Only that we be in its presence. That we fully, consciously hand ourselves over. That is all, and that is everything."

As a spiritual practice, surrender teaches us how to let go of small things in order to prepare us for the final giving over. Can we let go of a persistent thought or emotion, surrender to another's care when we'd prefer to care for ourselves, overlook a slight when our instinct is to point it out, choose to let go of the resentment that comes from not having our way? Learning to surrender can help all of us age with a greater sense of gratitude and grace. Jesus touches on this when speaking to Peter, who by nature was impetuous and willful. In telling Peter, he reminds all of us about the need for surrender, as things will be taken from us whether we like it or not:

> *Amen, amen I say to you, when you were younger, you used to dress yourself and go where you wanted; but when you grow old, you will stretch out your hands, and someone else will dress you and lead you where you do not want to go. – John 21:18*

Surrendering can gradually free us from the bonds of our own self-will and ego. In doing so we begin to peel back the layers of the false self to expose who we really are in God alone.

Begin by noticing the times you feel tense or anxious. There's a little illustrative exercise I do with people who are struggling with anxiety, pain, or loss. I hand them a pencil and ask them to clutch it as tightly as they can. In seconds they get tired. "Imagine grasping that pencil for hours, days, months, years? How would your hand feel?" Gratefully they put the pencil down. "Your fingers would ache, your arms would hurt, the tension and anxiety would intensify." They nod. The point is clear. Next I say, "Now squeeze the pencil as tightly as you can, then make a decision to release it." The point is you don't need to deny a feeling or your desire to respond in a negative way. Acknowledge and release. Name it, let it go. Hand it over to God. Tip the fulcrum toward the spirit self. You'll need to repeat the process multiple times, because the ego self will want to hold on. I always say, "Lord, I place this into your hands." Or, "I'm tired of carrying this – please take it." Repeat the phrase as needed. Remember – it's a *practice*. Start with little things and, gradually, move on to the more challenging.

What else to surrender? The obsessive wants that can dominate every moment of the day, the knee-jerk reactions, your typical responses, anything that might fall into the category of "That's just how I am" or "That's the way I do it." The process of sickness, dying, and death calls for a new perspective and will create a new reality.

Surrender is at the heart of all of the other practices – the necessary first step toward solitude, silence, and simplification.

SOLITUDE

Carving out time alone is essential to the spiritual life – the goal being to quiet the incessant *outside* noise. The scriptures reveal that seeking solitude, Jesus regularly retreated from the crowds and from his disciples.

> *Then he made the disciples get into the boat and precede him*
> *to the other side, while he dismissed the crowds. After doing*
> *this, he went up on the mountain by himself to pray.*

--MATTHEW 14:22-23

Yet, most of us tend to avoid solitude because we equate being alone with loneliness.

We live in a culture obsessed with noise and sensory overload. Restaurants have music playing, numerous TVs, each broadcasting a different sporting event. Patrons often have to shout in order to engage in conversation, thus raising the decibel level even more. Doctors' waiting rooms also have TVs; cars are equipped with speakers for radio and music, video screens so passengers can watch a movie. Even a walk or bike ride requires headphones, earbuds, ipod. Returning home, often the first reflexive move is to turn on the TV, providing an endless backdrop of noise and visual stimulation. This outer noise makes it almost impossible to embrace solitude.

When we do find ourselves alone, it can feel like an oppressive experience that touches into a primitive fear of mortality – an exaggerated perception of disconnectedness. So we build lives of frenetic activity, enabling us to skim the surface of life and relationships, creating the illusion of intimacy. Our sense of worth is derived from the things we do out in the world for others to see. A life continually lived outside oneself inhibits the ability to be reflective. It enables us to keep our inner lives (and our true selves) at bay. Because of this, embracing solitude is experienced as a threat to the false self.

It's interesting that the words solitude and solidarity both come from the Latin *solidum* – meaning 'whole sum'. They are also related to the Latin word for consolation and solace – *solari*. So, contrary to our perception of solitude as loneliness, the word is deeply rooted in the idea of consolation and solace as a sum of the whole. In sacred aloneness we experience *solidarity* with humanity, the world, and all of creation. Our Western culture continually tells us that we are distinct and unique from others, and holds this up as a value. This individualism can serve to isolate us in times of challenge as we try to handle a crisis on our own. The great surprise is that it is in solitude where we can begin to recognize that we are a part of everything and everyone - that we're all connected.

Catholic priest and author Henri Nouwen captures this in his book *Reaching Out:*

> "In this solitude we encourage each other to enter into the silence of our innermost being and discover the voice that calls us beyond the limits of human togetherness to a new communion. In this solitude we can slowly become aware of a presence of him who embraces friends and lovers and offers us the freedom to love each other, because he loved us first. (1 John 4: 19)"

The prayerful art of embracing solitude is crucial during sickness, dying, and death. While walking this Path of Suffering, you'll often find yourself alone. Your mobility may be limited, or your health may not allow you the freedom to leave the house as readily as you once did. As the world around you continues to turn, as family and friends go on with the responsibilities of their busy lives, you may find yourself on your own more often than you'd like. A stint at the hospital also involves a lot of alone time. Without loving intentionality, awareness, consent to embrace solitude, you'll experience an isolation in which the negative inner voices will flourish like bacteria in a petri dish.

So, how can you transform your potential loneliness and isolation into solitude?

- When you come into the house, resist the urge to turn on the TV, radio, or music. Turn off the ringer on your phone. Begin, instead, to be present and surrender to the moment. (As the Buddhists say, "When you're chopping wood, chop wood. When you're carrying water, carry water.") Resist the tendency to multi-task or to fast-forward to the future, or rewind to the past.
- Create a comfortable "alone" space. Include your favorite comfortable chair, good light, warm surroundings. Seek out this refuge on a regular basis. Instead of thinking of it as a lonely period, begin to think of it as privileged time shared with God alone.

SILENCE

When we embrace solitude, we consciously make an effort to avoid the outer noise that keeps us distracted. When I talk about silence, on the other hand, I'm talking about quieting the *inner* noise that prevents us from being still inside.

There is a strong relationship between solitude and silence. If we don't learn to cultivate solitude in our aloneness, we'll experience great loneliness. This is when the inner noise – the bullying self talk, self-recrimination, and anxious chatter – creep in and begin to dominate. It prohibits mindfulness, blocks inner reflection, and feeds the 'barking dogs' of worry and anxiety raging inside. It also diminishes relational intimacy. This is where, once again, awareness, intention, and consent come in.

Once we're aware of the connection between solitude (retreating from outside noise) and silence (calming the inner noise), we can intentionally surrender our seemingly innate need for auditory clutter, seeking out places of quiet. Then I introduce people to the "walking stick" or sacred mantra. I'm always reminded of the twenty third Psalm:

> *Even when I walk through a dark valley, I fear no harm for you are at my side; your rod and staff give me courage.*

The "rod and staff" that can give you courage is the 'walking stick'. When 68 year old Joe's heart was failing he found himself in the hospital over and over again. "I dreaded the nights," he said. "Could never sleep. The beeping of the monitors drove me crazy. I was always listening to the rhythm, waiting for the skip that would indicate my heart had had enough. The more I obsessed on it, the more anxiety I'd feel. Then I'd worry that my anxiety would trigger another heart attack. It was a vicious cycle."

I introduced Joe to the use of the "walking stick," a simple word or phrase that anchors your intention in God. It might be, *"Jesus, my love,"* or *"I thirst for you."* Any snippet of scripture or a personal invitation to God. Joe learned to offer his consent to God's presence, to invite God into the situation, and to use his short mantra to help draw his attention away from the internal and external noise that was stealing precious minutes of life from him.

"As soon as the anxiety started I'd use my walking stick," Joe said. *I fear no harm, for you are at my side...* I'd repeat it until I believed it. Until I felt a calming presence. With that calm came a deep joy, because I knew it was God, right there with me."

Here's how to engage in silence as an intentional practice:

- Become mindful of the ways we continually block out and avoid silence. The constant noise and stimulation can become a crutch for blocking out the inner voices that torment us.
- Instead of trying to drown out the inner voices, the goal is to roll them out, acknowledge them, then gently let them go. (This is the basis for meditation or centering prayer.)
- Find a quiet place of solitude, and acknowledge and consent to God's presence within you. Removing these distractions will, at first, open the floodgates for negative internal chatter. But, indulging or suppressing these voices only gives them more power.

Virginia, my friend and parishioner, gets up a half an hour earlier than she needs to. She lights a small candle and sits, in silence, at the kitchen table. Another parishioner uses her car as a silent refuge. It took a little practice not to immediately reach for the radio, but driving, which is largely a right brain, intuitive activity, is well suited to a silent practice. Still others enjoy the quiet sounds of nature available in their backyards, or a walk by the shore or along a forest trail. Whatever quiet sanctuary you choose, the key is to acknowledge the fertile patch inside where God and the True Self coexist, and to simply "be" there. The consent to and practice of silence goes hand-in-hand with solitude.

So, begin slowly and with intention.

As you consciously create silence, what do you notice? Does the silence press in and make you anxious? If so, good! It's a sign that the false self is threatened. You're removing some of the stimulation that the false self thrives on that masks the true self. Sit in it and observe. You can commit to this in your car as well. Invite God into the car with you. Invite your true self to become your navigator.

SIMPLIFICATION

As we move through the phases of sickness, dying and death our lives become more complicated. Even basic day-to-day activities can be challenging, necessitating all kinds of modifications to accommodate this new ever-changing reality. Life isn't normal anymore, and as our world seems to grow smaller, the tiniest details within it become larger.

This necessitates a move toward simplification. Letting go of expectations about what normal is. Getting down to basics. Detachment. During the final years of my dad's life, as he became less and less independent, he used to say, "Tommy, don't sweat the small stuff... and what's small stuff now is stuff I used to think was pretty important."

But, there's another dimension of simplification beyond what is dictated by our decreased ability to deal with the practical demands of living. On a spiritual level, simplification can be defined as *single-heartedness*. To simplify spiritually means to narrow our focus from worldly concerns to Godly concerns, to spend whatever energy we have in the work of loving. Nurturing relationships. Expressing gratitude. Forgiving and reconciling. As your energy wanes all else can fall by the wayside, and it comes down to one simple thing – your ability to love. Jesus points to this in the Beatitudes (Matthew 5:8) when he says, *"Blessed are the clean of heart, for they will see God."* Think of simplification as reducing your life to its very essence. Begin giving "stuff" away. Things you once saw as important and now see for what they are – clutter which threatens solitude and silence. With increasingly limited time and energy it's important to reserve your emotional resources for what's most important –being open to be filled to overflowing with God's love.

Simplification is closely tied to surrender, as it involves letting go of anything that distracts us from the single-hearted attention to and intention of loving. It also goes hand in hand with solitude. Henri Nouwen, in his book *Reaching Out* speaks to this:

"Without solitude of heart, our relationships with others easily become needy and greedy, sticky and clinging, dependent and sentimental, exploitative and parasitic, because without the solitude of heart we cannot experience the others as different from ourselves but only as people who can be used for the fulfillment of our own, often hidden, needs."

THE INTERPLAY OF THE FOUR "S" PRACTICES

Embracing the art of surrender, solitude, silence, and simplification can, during "the green times," bring a richness and depth to our lives that is far more satisfying than the passing pleasures the world offers. During the challenges of sickness and dying these practices are even more important. We learn not to take things too seriously, to put our frustration into perspective, and to be gentle with ourselves and others. During the process of an illness, for both the patient and the caregiver, the four "S" practices can become the lifeline that keeps them afloat, one day (or one hour) at a time. When emotions flare, when the inner voices drive you crazy, when you feel that "enough is enough" you can acknowledge all of it without fueling the flames and fanning the fire. Through the four S practices, we build a firm foundation for the spiritual practices we'll explore in the next chapter.

CHAPTER 17

Spiritual Practices - Empty and Fill

"My grace is sufficient for you, for power is made perfect in weakness."

-- 2 Corinthians 12:9

WHAT DID JESUS mean in these words to St. Paul? And what is the significance for us, especially during the process of sickness and dying? It is at the heart of what I call "Empty, Fill, and Spill." When we're depleted by our suffering (empty), a space is created in which we allow God's love to grow (fill). As we become more and more open to this love, when we're filled to the brim with it, it overflows onto everyone and everything we touch (spill). This love that pours from our emptiness is the purest of all love, as it flows through us directly from God.

A wonderful symbol of this dynamic comes from the prophet Ezekiel:

Then he brought me back to the entrance of the temple, and there I saw water flowing out from beneath the threshold of the temple toward the east, for the facade of the temple was toward the east; the water flowed down from the southern side of the temple, south of the altar. He led me outside by the north gate, and around to the outer gate facing the east, where I saw water trickling from the southern side. Then when he had walked off to the east with a measuring cord in his hand, he measured off a thousand cubits and had me wade through the water, which was ankle-deep. He measured off another thousand and once more had me wade through the water, which

*was now knee deep. Again he measured off a thousand and had me
wade; the water was up to my waist. Once more he measured off a
thousand, but there was now a river through which I could not wade;
for the water had risen so high it had become a river that could not
be crossed except by swimming. He asked me, "Have you seen this,
son of man? " Then he brought me to the bank of the river, where
he had me sit. Along the bank of the river I saw very many trees on
both sides. He said to me, "This water flows into the eastern district
down upon the Arabah, and empties into the sea, the salt waters,
which it makes fresh. Wherever the water flows, every sort of living
creature that can multiply shall live, and there shall be abundant
fish, for wherever this water comes the sea shall be made fresh. Along
both banks of the river fruit trees of every kind shall grow; their
leaves shall not fade nor their fruit fail. Every month they shall bear
fresh fruit for they shall be watered by the flow from the sanctuary.
Their fruit shall serve for food, and their leaves for medicine."*

-- EZEKIEL: 47:1-9, 12

Where these waters flow, they refresh... Ezekiel speaks of the temple metaphorically. We are all temples of God into and from which living waters
flow that can heal and refresh. In 1Corinthians 6:19 St. Paul writes:

*"Do you not know that your body is the temple of the Holy Spirit within
you, whom you have from God, and that you are not your own? "*

This image of the temple being filled with water to overflowing – first as
a trickle, then ankle deep, waist deep, and finally overflowing, producing a fertile field - what a perfect image of **"Empty, Fill, and Spill."**

Not only are the spiritual practices designed to maximize the
"Empty" and "Fill" part of this process, but they are, in a sense, a spiritual and emotional rehearsal that helps prepare us for what we'll face
in the handing over of our own lives – in our loving, our suffering, and
in our dying. The practices deepen your awareness of the working of

God in your life, helping you to understand that you are and always have been loved by God, and out of this sense of wholeness you can begin to live out of this love. Another gift is that, over time, they transform an intellectual understanding that "I am loved by God" into a deep knowing. This profound, core experience of God's love creates an openness that allows you to become an instrument of that love that you will share with others. The four practices I share with you are: **Praying the Everyday, Fasting from Negativity, Meditation,** and **Lectio Divina.** My hope is that as you engage in these practices, you'll experience God's love in a greater way and begin to see the fruits of His love being poured out on all those you encounter.

"EVERYDAY PRAYER" AND "PRAYING THE EVERYDAY"

Theologian Karl Rahner, S.J. wrote a book titled: *The Need and the Blessing of Prayer.* The year was 1946, the place, Munich, which had been largely destroyed during the war. Amidst the rubble and devastation Rahner addressed a people who had been diminished by suffering and loss.

Fr. Rahner spoke about the power of prayer. He distinguished between what he called "everyday prayer" and "praying the everyday." Most of us are familiar with everyday prayer - the well-known prayers of our childhood that we recite, prayers before meals, at rising and at bedtime. Prayers of petition, expressing our needs and desires to God. All of these initiate an openness to the God within. They can be thought of as the first trickle of "filling" the self with God's love.

While these everyday prayers can "prime the pump" they can easily become prayers of duty and custom. Still, Rahner explains, everyday prayers are important – they do, to some extent, keep God on our radar. The problem is, in times of great challenge we can experience a disconnect between the words we express and our inner emotional landscape. The words of faith, of thanksgiving, or repentance cease to ring true when juxtaposed over the fear, resentment, and sorrow that dominates the situation we find ourselves in. Even in the best of times,

Rahner warns of "routinizing prayer." It can, he says, "become exterior, mechanical, heartless, lip-prayer."

This is why Fr. Rahner advocated for "praying the everyday." He describes the everydayness of life, the often thankless efforts we invest in work and in relationships, the failures and disappointments we struggle through, and the unrequited dreams we're forced to let go of. How can the mundaneness of life possibly bring us into a greater awareness of God? This takes us back to the disposition of surrender. Rahner explains that the very stuff of life, if embraced, can teach us to die to ourselves a little each day. As this small incremental dying occurs, something else is happening, if we have the eyes to see it – the rising of love. Put more simply, the most powerful prayer is when we can, in God's name and power, dedicate all to God, offering up our everyday, whatever it brings, as our prayer. And, it comes back again to fulcrum, as Rahner explains,

"Only in this way does it (life) serve the love of God, for only so does it take us away from ourselves. If we let ourselves be taken by the everyday, our longing, our self-assertion, our obstinacy, our walled-in ourselfness, that is, if we don't become bitter in our bitterness, ordinary in our ordinariness, everyday in our every-dayness, disappointed in our disappointment, if we let ourselves be educated through the everyday to kindness, to patience, to peace and understanding, to forbearance and meekness, to for-giveness and endurance, to selfless loyalty, then everyday is no longer everyday, then it is prayer."

This "praying the everyday" requires awareness, intention, consent, and practice as well as a daily renewal of these dispositions. It is a movement to radical inclusiveness, that all – the good, the bad, the pain, the joy, the full range of human feelings, emotions, and experiences – that all become an expression of the one life we're given here, and thus offered, as sacred, back to God. This is what it means to "Pray the Everyday." There is no greater prayer that we can offer.

During sickness, dying, and death "praying the everyday" might be all we have the strength to do. I'm reminded of my friend Phil, at the brink of death, raising a glass of scotch in a small toast, proclaiming, "What can I say? Here I am Lord." Praying the everyday. Proclaiming the ordinary holy.

FASTING (*REMOVING THE BRAMBLE FROM THE FIELD OF YOUR HEART.*)

An age-old and often misunderstood spiritual practice is *fasting*. In the early days of the church Christians believed that by refraining from or limiting what they ate they would feed the soul by denying the body (referred to as "mortification of the flesh"). This represented a "death" to the many human appetites that often led to self-absorption and sin. In more recent times Christians are encouraged to abstain from eating certain foods on designated days of the week and during different liturgical seasons, such as Lent.

However, Jesus, in response to questions about the lack of fasting among his disciples, addresses the heart of the matter in Matthew 15:11, saying,

> *"It is not what enters one's mouth that defiles that person; but what comes out of the mouth is what defiles one."*

Jesus understood that there are more important forms of fasting. Some forms of fasting require a greater level of "letting go" than others. I tell my parishioners every Lent not to worry about giving up chocolate, or that nightly glass of wine, or whatever else they try to white-knuckle through Lent in order to demonstrate their willpower and righteousness (and often, lose a few unwanted pounds in the process). Instead I ask them to fast from what Jesus refers to as "what proceeds out of the mouth" – what I call the **negative relational behaviors.** When we're snarky, chippy, demanding, complaining, or outright confrontational we create an atmosphere of tension, resentment, and negativity that

180

initiates an ongoing cycle of hurt. These negative relational behaviors are all rooted in the ego self (the false self) and tend to be our unintentional, automatic response when we're threatened. Think about it: we don't plan ways to lash out at those we love and care for – it's reactive rather than proactive behavior. We don't have to "practice the negative behaviors" – they just seem to happen. It's so emotionally driven by any threat to the ego that we aren't able to consider the consequences. When we're tired or depleted, self-absorbed with worry and anxiety, our level of defensiveness and irritability can skyrocket. The result is that, in varying degrees, we hurt everyone who crosses our path. And those nearest and dearest are generally the bull's eye on the target.

As we move along the Path of Suffering it's important to be aware of this dynamic, and to intentionally ask for God's help in breaking the cycle of negative relational behaviors. Doing so amounts to cutting back the invasive thorns and bramble that can quickly overrun the sacred field of your heart. See if any of these behaviors, below, are familiar.

WHEN THREATENED WE BECOME:

- Preoccupied
- Negative
- Critical
- Self-Absorbed
- Mistrustful
- Judgmental

- Emotionally Withdrawn
- Rejecting
- Ungrateful
- Resistant
- Insensitive
- Discouraging

- Indifferent
- Abusive
- Demanding
- Uncooperative
- Punitive
- Sarcastic

No one wants to think of themselves in these terms, and I don't mention them in order to lay Catholic Guilt on you or to have you indulge in a pity party. Awareness is the first step toward any positive change. Your intention to fast from negative behaviors will open your heart to consent to God's prompting and grace. It is only in and through God's love that you'll be able to interrupt this natural tendency to lash out or to withdraw. Surrendering yourself to become a vessel of God's love will quiet the ego, and create a buffer for the vulnerability you feel so bent on defending. As you become free enough to let go in this way you'll gradually see a more positive relational climate – and it's only in a warm, trusting environment that we can engage in the many loving encounters and conversations that need to take place in order to leave this world with a sense of peace, hope, joy, and love.

Fasting from negative behaviors is like removing the bramble and thorns from the soil of your heart. This is the first step toward expanding the fertile patch of your soul into a verdant field.

Keep the list of negative behaviors before you. Look at it as you begin the day and pray for God's help. It is God's strength that becomes our courage, without which we cannot really do anything that is life-giving. Notice how it feels when you "let go and let God," choosing love and kindness over angst and resentment. When you do, you can begin to see, concretely, the working of God in your life. The fruits are the evidence. This "letting go and letting God," in itself, becomes a spiritual practice that will open you up to the important work still to come – doing little things with great love, telling your story to others, forgiving those who've hurt you, and being vulnerable enough to express gratitude and say your goodbyes.

And when you fail, as you inevitably will, apologize. Ask for forgiveness. But don't beat yourself up. You're only human. Get up and start again, more humble, more compassionate, more reliant on God, and more aware of the freedom that comes with choosing the most loving response. This is why we call it a *practice* - because we never get it right the first time.

MEDITATION AND LECTIO DIVINA

Meditation and Lectio Divina are two classic practices that can draw us closer to God, helping to quiet the inner voices that can dominate our consciousness. These practices deflect us from our obsessive focus on self, creating an inner space that can be filled with God.

If you begin these practices in "the green times" of life unimpeded by the challenges of serious sickness or caregiving you can embrace the whole of the process as laid out for you here. Also, there are many books solely devoted to each of these, which you can explore to enrich and deepen your practice.

Those approaching these practices for the first time, who find themselves on the Path of Suffering, may need to make some modifications due to the physical and emotional limitations inherent in the dying process. I'll suggest some modifications that many have found helpful and I encourage you to adapt these practices based on your own individual situation.

Whatever your ability to carry out these practices, your awareness, intention, and consent to God will bear fruit. The key is to be gentle with yourself, and recommit to your practice daily.

MEDITATION

There are many methods of meditation, but I'll describe the practice known as Centering Prayer or contemplation. Meditation has often been touted as a tool for relaxation and wellness, and it is. But it is *so* much more than that.

First, it's important to dispel some of the misconceptions people have about meditation. To the uninitiated, it may seem that the goal of meditation is to put the mind into a static state, dispelling thoughts and holding them at arm's length, shutting down the brain for awhile – a little like placing a computer in sleep mode. While the possibility of controlling negative thoughts and anxiety may sound appealing, the truth is that there is no way to tether our thoughts. Meditation is more about acknowledging, honoring, and letting go of our thoughts and emotions so that *they don't control us.*

We also don't meditate in order to engage in deep thinking about God, to look for some personal sign, insight, or message, but rather *to simply be with God.* In the context of seasoned, mature faith, we begin to realize that God is greater than our intellect, a mystery more expansive than we can grasp through thoughts or express via language. As soon as we begin to feel that we totally "get it," all we've really done is shrink God down to our size. Instead, in meditation, we approach God with all our sensibilities open, with a willingness to accept and experience a God that we acknowledge is beyond the limits of our capacities. We begin to understand that God is both within us and others, present in the moment, and at the same time light years beyond us. The only way we can begin to experience this unfathomable paradox of God is through a deep, still silence. This is reflected in Psalm 46:11: *Be still and know that I am God!*

Many have forgotten that meditation has always been an important part of the Christian tradition. When Jesus talked about prayer, instructing his disciples to "retreat to their inner room" he was asking them to meditate:

> *But you, when you pray, go into your inner room, close the door, and pray to your Father in secret. And your Father who sees in secret will repay you. In praying, do not babble like the pagans, who think that they will be heard because of their many words. Do not be like them, for your Father knows what you need before you ask him. –Matthew 6:7*

The desert fathers, mothers, and mystics of the church (John of the Cross, Julian of Norwich, Theresa of Avila, Saint Teresa of Calcutta, among scores of others) all deepened their faith and had profound experiences of God through meditation. In their writings they tell us that, over time, a meditative practice helps the practitioner to intuitively know God (as opposed to knowing *about* God) – and that's a huge difference.

Surrender, silence, and solitude are the building blocks of meditation. But, unlike what we generally think of as prayer, meditation is geared toward emptying and *listening*. It's about *receptivity* rather than petitioning, about carving out a space where *God* can speak – not necessarily in words, but in ways that mysteriously touch the deepest recesses of our souls. A meditative practice peels back the many layers of the ego, so that we begin to recognize ourselves as who we are in God alone – in other words, we slowly and gradually learn to embrace our true selves and open ourselves to God's loving presence within.

HOW TO BEGIN MEDITATION OR CENTERING PRAYER

- Find a quiet spot where you can sit comfortably.
- Close your eyes for a moment and offer God your consent. The words don't need to be formulaic or fancy. You might simply say, *"God, I open my heart to your presence."* Or, *"I consent to your presence within me."*
- Set the timer on your phone, watch, or other device for five minutes. Close your eyes. Enter into the silence. Feel it as something tangible – the thickness and substance of it. Gradually, increase the time you spend in quiet meditation to 20 minutes, and eventually 20 minutes twice a day.
- Choose your sacred word. Your sacred word or phrase, might be: *"Jesus,"* or, *"I thirst."*
- As thoughts begin to traipse through your brain (as they surely will) gently acknowledge them and let them go. It's a little like watching fish in an aquarium – you see them, then they swim past. Don't try to catch them, analyze them, or obsess on them. *The goal isn't to try to stop the thoughts – that's impossible – the goal is to release them.* In Fr. Joseph Langford's book, *Mother Theresa's Secret Fire*, he compares the practice of meditation to someone diving for pearls. The diver descends into the depths to begin the search. Deeper, deeper, but occasionally he floats toward the surface. When that happens the diver will gently kick with his flippers to submerge again. He repeats this and eventually captures the pearl of great price. Meditation is like that – we go deep into our inner room, but often distractions

bring us to the surface. That's when we give a gentle kick and plunge to the depths again. You may also become aware of the rhythm of your breathing, slow and steady, consciously inhaling the Spirit of God, exhaling all you hold on to that blocks God's presence.

- Use your sacred word (the metaphorical "kick of the flipper") that helps you return to the deep. When your thoughts begin to dominate, gently repeat your sacred word. Doing so restates your intention and consent, and redirects your attention to the silence you're embracing. When you first try meditation don't be surprised if you need to repeat your sacred phrase *continually*. This becomes your sacred mantra, constantly reaffirming your intention.

After a month or so of consistent practice you'll find yourself drawn to it, even looking forward to it, though you likely won't be able to name the reasons why. You become a little freer, the voices inside a little less strident, the feelings less oppressive. It's not that you've conquered your thoughts and feelings, but that you've learned the freedom that comes from *surrendering them*. Your meditation has become a quiet discipline that, without you realizing it, has been continually and consistently expanding the fertile patch, clearing a pathway for God.

Your sacred word can also be used in times when you feel alone, anxious, sad or angry - surrendering the feelings and focusing instead on your oneness with God. When Linda, one of my parishioners, underwent a serious surgery for complications from cancer, she used her sacred words (what I call a "walking stick") to draw herself into God's embrace as she was prepped for the procedure, wheeled to the operating room, right up until the moment anesthesia was administered. She used a line from Psalm 16: *Keep me safe, O my God, in you I take refuge.* "Throughout the whole ordeal I was one with God," she said. "I was never afraid – not of pain, and not of death. God was a gentle presence there beside me the entire time."

One common question is, "What if I fall asleep while meditating?" Sometimes during meditation my steady breathing shifts to a soft snore. My dear friend, Father Carl Arico of Contemplative Outreach has said to me, "Tom, what makes you think God loves you any less when you're asleep? " Consent to slumbering in the arms of God if that's where your meditation brings you.

> **Modification:** For patients farther along in the dying process, or those struggling with debilitating pain, I try to stress the importance of the "walking stick" or sacred. Repeating a sacred phrase can ease the anxiety and focus the attention away from the ego self and onto God. And it can be a foundational stepping stone to meditation. (For more information and resources on Centering Prayer, go to www.**contemplativeoutreach**.org.)

LECTIO DIVINA

Lectio Divina (literally, "Divine reading") is a contemplative approach to reading and understanding Sacred Scripture. Anyone who has attended religious services of any denomination has likely heard God's Word proclaimed to the congregation. Often we listen to the words, but never really hear them. We might perceive the scriptures as holy cautionary tales or as God's rulebook handed down through the generations. Or we might appreciate the ancient texts as one might enjoy poetry from a bygone era.

But the sacred texts of all traditions, regardless of when they were written, are actually living, breathing documents that possess the power to speak personally to regular people across the ages. While the overall themes are timeless, and, at face value, provide a set of values and moral teachings that a given religion subscribes to, the Word of God is intended to be so much more.

Indeed, the word of God is living and effective, sharper than any two edged sword, penetrating even between soul and spirit, joints and marrow, and able to discern reflections and thoughts of the heart. – Hebrews 4:12

In the Christian tradition the Bible presents us with a fascinating study of the nature of God and of humanity, and the relationship between the two. It validates our struggles and provides us with hope in the promises God has made to God's people.

The practice of Lectio Divina opens our ears and our hearts to understand the unique message from God for us that's alive in the Scriptures. Instead of listening as an objective third party, or as a scholar might analyze and critique a text for literal or historical content, we begin by offering our memories and insecurities, hopes and worries to our God – in other words, we engage from a place of vulnerability. As in any relationship, when we expose ourselves in this way, and approach the encounter openly and honestly, we build intimacy. We become more receptive, taking in each word, picking up on the multitude of ways that the message in the sacred text applies to us individually and uniquely at that particular point in our journeys. The words touch us personally, as does any loving conversation. Certain phrases suddenly resonate, revealing something new about God and self. We become filled with God's presence, communicated through God's word.

How to Begin Lectio Divina

- Choose a passage of Scripture to read and reflect on. I always prefer to select the daily readings designated by the Catholic Church, knowing that, over time, I'll be exposed to a good portion of the Bible. (The readings are organized in three-year cycles, with a different collection of Old and New Testament excerpts each day.) I have a free app on my phone called **Laudate** that provides these daily readings. From their menu I choose "Daily Readings and Saint of the Day." This calls up an Old Testament reading, a Psalm, and a New Testament (Gospel) reading. I usually select the Psalm or Gospel reading for my Lectio practice. But, you can use any sacred text.

Another favorite app is called *iMissal*. It offers the option to hear the scripture read aloud.

- Find a comfortable, quiet place to sit and settle yourself, as you do when meditating. You may use your "walking stick" – your sacred word or phrase, to still your inner distractions.

- Offer God your consent and intention. You might say something like, "God open my ears and my heart to your words for me today." I always think of the story in the Old Testament where God appears to Samuel and Samuel says: *Speak, for your servant is listening. – 1 Samuel 3:10*

- Read your selected passage slowly. I always recommend reading it aloud. It's important for the word to be *proclaimed.* Reading aloud also allows us to actually *hear* the words, which we perceive very differently than words read silently. Seeing the words, speaking them, and hearing them, simultaneously, is a multisensory experience. Be aware of any word, phrase, or image that resonates or stands out. You don't need to try to figure out why it moves you – just quietly accept that the word, phrase, or image carries some personal relevance. You might think of this resonance as an invitation from God to better understand yourself, and your relationship with God and others.

- Gently read the passage a second time, asking what the message is for you. Pay special attention to the resounding word or phrase, or see the image more closely. Allow it to conjure up memories, stir up concerns, to intermingle with the deepest parts of yourself. Ponder these connections, understanding that God wants to be a part of your inner world. The word, phrase, or image will likely arouse, challenge or validate some aspect of yourself, affirming that God is present and caring at this seminal level. Sit quietly in this experience, letting it wash over and fill you.

- Read the passage a third time, with an ear for what God would like you to do with the insight you've received. Feel free to speak to God in response to this. If you're unclear about the message, ask for clarity. Don't expect instant answers or lightning bolts of understanding. Rather, carry the word, phrase, or image into your day with a sense of expectant hope, and faith that the significance will eventually reveal itself to you. This might be a time where you wrestle with God. For example, I can think of days when the message I received was not one I particularly wanted to hear. I would be honest and forthcoming; my prayer would be, *"Lord, I'm not ready for this. I'm afraid. Help me, please."* Getting in touch with these kinds of feelings and expressing them can be very freeing and grace-filled, trusting that God will respond by either resolving the situation or giving you unfailing strength to stand in it. Always return to your word, phrase, or image. You might jot it down daily in a journal, commit it to memory, keeping it there for the ready. As you revisit and reflect on it, it will begin to inform and transform some aspect of your life.

- Finally, rest in the word, phrase, or image you received from sacred scripture. Turn it over gently in your mind, then let it go, allowing it to permeate the deepest parts of your soul, to become a part of you.

Personally, I often approach Lectio through what is called "imaginative reading." I picture myself as part of the scene described, as one of the characters in the story, or as a bystander observing what's taking place. For example, if reading the story of the Prodigal Son (Luke 15:11-32) I might assume the point of view of the merciful father, the resentful son, or the prodigal son. I try to understand this character's response, try and identify the hurts he must have suffered. In other words, I walk in another character's shoes, with compassion. I observe how their actions affect me, notice what my knee-jerk responses are. And finally, I carry this character out of the text and into my heart in order to see how we are the same, or different, and what that says about my faith.

Modification: Select a shorter passage. If you lack the energy or ability to read the word, invite someone to read it to you or use one of the apps mentioned earlier. Marge, one of my parishioners, had her son write her word or phrase on a large piece of paper and tape it to the wall opposite her bed. In this way she could return to it throughout the day. It was the first thing she saw in the morning, and the last thing before sleep at night. It became an anchor for her, keeping her from drifting into fear, worry, self-absorption.

You might ask whether or not any insight or message received is truly from God, or simply your own inner voice. I always ask myself one question as a means of discerning God's word from my own; is the message and meaning rooted deeply in love? If so, I trust that it is of God.

Linking a meditative practice with Lectio Divina is a powerful combination – an example of "empty" and "fill." You empty yourself through meditation, then fill yourself with the Word of God. Pope Benedict spoke of this:

> "Diligent reading of Sacred Scripture accompanied by prayer brings about that intimate dialogue in which the person reading hears God who is speaking, and in praying, responds to him with trusting openness of heart." (cf. Dei Verbum 25).

Barbara begins each day with meditation, followed by Lectio Divina. On days when work takes her on the road, and her morning schedule makes this routine impossible there's a radically different texture and tone to her day. Everything feels more harried and hurried. Small frustrations become larger than they need to be. Persistent negative thoughts and self-talk can begin to dominate. Barbara says, "While it might seem difficult to make time for the practice, *not* practicing is so much harder."

Lectio Divina can also be a meaningful group practice. Check with your church community to see if there are any groups near you – or form one with trusted friends or family members. Having the same scripture read aloud by different voices also adds another dimension to the practice. It's fascinating to see how others are moved by different aspects of the same reading. These insights can be expansive and enlightening. Sharing not only builds intimacy with God, but with neighbor as well.

FROM ACCEPTANCE TO TRANSFORMATION

The spiritual practices are vehicles for moving toward, and hopefully beyond, acceptance. Much has been written about acceptance as the doorway to a peaceful death. And it's true – once you accept your place on the Path of Suffering, understand that your own turn to die is approaching, and you decide that enough is enough, the voices in your head and the anxiety you wrestle with throughout each day will begin to recede. Acceptance is a positive alternative to resignation (which is usually steeped in negativity and bitterness). Medicine can alleviate much of the physical pain associated with the body shutting down, and accepting your fate can reduce any mental anguish or emotional suffering. It's a relief to be able to give up the fight and begin a peaceful time of vigil.

Transformation, on the other hand, is not as much about inner peace during the winding down phase (although inner peace is a by-product of transformation) as it is about reaching out of an increasingly fragile self *unconditionally*, allowing yourself to become a channel for the purity and power of God's love. A person can come to acceptance and still be rooted firmly in the ego self. The focus is still on control, although perhaps in a more subtle way.

Transformation weds your true self to God and all of creation. It is about becoming free from the shackles of the ego, and with that new freedom bursts an astonishing ability to love out of your suffering. Transformation is the process of handing everything over to God and resting in God's unconditional love, forgiveness, and healing. When it happens you realize you already have one foot in heaven and you suddenly understand that you *always have!* The whole generative thrust of transformation drives us out of ourselves to bring joy and love to others. It is about renewal. Recreation of self *and others*. It is about expanding our ability to love, by emptying ourselves and becoming ever more receptive vessels, eager to carry and share God's unconditional love and mercy in a broken world.

That's what the rest of this book is about.

CHAPTER 18

Communal Worship - Being Filled with God's Intimate Love

WHY WE WORSHIP

OVER THE YEARS, I've come to believe that within all of us there's a need to worship someone or something greater than ourselves to help us deal with the challenges of life. Some hold up a lifestyle, others immerse themselves in an activity, still others lose themselves in a relationship.

Some choose to worship their God. Pope Francis speaks of these choices:

> "When we do not adore God, we adore something else. Money and power are false idols which often take the place of God."

I know Pope Francis is right. What I've seen in dealing with suffering is that the only life-giving focus that gets us out of our own way is a profound and personal encounter with the living God. Facilitating this sacred encounter is a primary function of both spiritual practices and communal worship. Whatever your religious tradition, gathering to worship provides a means to communicate with God through ritual, symbol, prayer, and song. Regardless of the denomination, time and space is set aside for sacred rituals designed to create an opportunity for worshippers to open their hearts to mystery. The formal use of prescribed movement, traditional words, symbolic objects, the sights, sounds, and smells encourage participants to satisfy their deepest longings and desires by having a personal interaction with God. As Carl Jung believed, symbols are the best possible expression for something unknown. In other words, the rich symbols evident in religious rituals evoke a deep "knowing" of truths beyond what we can articulate. Therefore, no matter what religious tradition you hold, never underestimate the power of your worship.

Often, I hear people evaluating their particular religious services in terms of how engaging they are (or aren't.) Whether the homily was meaningful, the music stimulating, the clergy and congregants welcoming, the environment pleasing. Of course, if all of this passes muster, so much the better. But, if it doesn't (and, because all places of worship are comprised of fallible humans, our services are *never* perfect) *the imperfections cannot diminish the underlying power of what draws us to mystery in the first place.* In Catholic worship, congregants are fed at the Lord's table during the breaking and sharing of the bread, and nourished by the proclamation of God's Word. These ancient rituals, established by Jesus himself, draw people back, again and again, as they have for centuries.

I always urge parishioners to come and participate in worship in a full, active, and conscious way. Communal worship calls us to reflect on how God's love has been manifested in our lives and the lives of others. The recognition of what God has done for us in the past, is doing for us now, and God's promises for the future inspire us to praise and thank God. Congregants are encouraged to engage in hospitable fellowship, active participation, reverential silence, all with an attitude of love toward one another. Worship also stirs us to respond with a resounding "yes" to God's ongoing invitation: *Will you let me love you?* This "yes" opens our hearts to God's gifts of love, forgiveness, and healing that already exist within each of us – we just fail to see them. Worship can help us open our eyes to God's gifts so that we can experience a sense of oneness with God, with others, and with all that is.

THE INTERPLAY BETWEEN SPIRITUAL PRACTICES AND WORSHIP

Remember the Prophet Ezekiel's Scripture passage in the last chapter about the water flowing from the temple? How it started gradually and expanded until it overflowed the riverbanks, and all that was watered grew and bore fruit? Similarly, as we open our hearts through individual spiritual practices we begin to water our faith.

Worship, however, is rooted in community. The stream that waters our faith flows through all who come together to worship. Our awareness of the Indwelling, honed through individual spiritual practice, expands exponentially as we begin to recognize the gift of God within the *other*. With this recognition comes the insight that we're not only coming together to offer praise and thanksgiving to our God, or to pursue a personal encounter with God, but we gather together to better experience and honor the indwelling of God in those who we worship with. Through eyes of faith we're able to see God in others, even when hidden in a variety of unique disguises. Every person has a story, every one of us is broken in some way. All share a deep longing to be loved, and a need for God's unconditional love and mercy. Something powerful happens when a community begins to recognize this, all standing together before this great mystery. There is something Trinitarian in the dynamic of God, self, and neighbor that happens during worship if we're open to it. As we hear in Matthew 18:20: *Where two or three are gathered together in my name, there am I in the midst of them.*

THE BENEFITS OF WORSHIP DURING SICKNESS AND DYING

Amelia was a parishioner at St. James, a quiet, gentle woman, and a regular attendee at the 7:30 Sunday morning mass. Around the time of her 60th birthday she was diagnosed with cervical cancer. As her short brown curls thinned and were replaced by a turban, as her already willowy frame became even thinner, the 7:30 community was there to support her. Though a private person, who engaged in a number of spiritual practices at home, Amelia continued coming to mass, and graciously accepted the words of encouragement, the prayers, and the offers of every kind of practical assistance, sometimes from people she barely knew.

"There are days when I just want to stay home," Amelia had said. "But, as everything in my life is changing, I'm comforted by the fact that mass is always the same, that everyone here – even those I don't know – are all here for the same reason. There's a timelessness about this rite that's been performed in faith, through the centuries. As so much of who I am seems lost, coming here makes me feel a part of something greater. Like I'm not going through this alone."

For sure, communal worship can be a balm for a patient or caregiver who comes to the table with nothing to offer but their empty selves. This was certainly the case with Amelia, and countless others. Those who are suffering can ride the wave of this blessedly familiar movement toward mystery and be buoyed by it. As Amelia faced the unknown, moving closer to the threshold of death, the more deeply and reverently she entered the ritual and embraced the mysteries inherent in it. Doing so served as a rehearsal for the greatest mystery of all - her own dying.

WORSHIP THROUGH THE CATHOLIC CHRISTIAN LENS

In the Catholic Church, we refer to our communal gathering as the *liturgy,* as do many other denominations. Liturgy is often defined as "the work of the people." I always remind my congregation that the priest isn't celebrating the mass for them – he's presiding over a celebration in which we all work together to help each other open a pathway to God.

For those of other faith traditions: As we look at the Eucharist, please consider the symbols, structure, and traditions of your communal worship and how your ritual celebrations open the hearts of its members to encounter the living God and then send them forth to share God's love with others.

THE EUCHARIST

The Catholic liturgy is made up of two major movements – the Liturgy of the Word and the Liturgy of the Eucharist. (The ritual in its entirety is also referred to as the Eucharist.) Listen to this section of one of the

Eucharistic prayers which points to these two movements and the way they're rooted in God's steadfast love for us:

> *You are indeed Holy and to be glorified, O God,*
> *who loves the human race,*
> *and who always walks with us on the journey of life.*
> *Blessed indeed is your Son,*
> *present in our midst when we are gathered by his love,*
> *and when, as once for the disciples, so now for us,*
> **he opens the scripture and breaks the bread.**

LITURGY OF THE WORD

The Liturgy of the Word consists of the reading of Sacred Scripture. When the Scripture is read aloud, it's important to understand that The Word is not static, but *living and active*. We tend to think of the "real presence" of God in the breaking of the bread at communion time, but often forget that God's real presence is also revealed in the proclamation of The Word. Instead of thinking of the Scripture as an account of a past event, listen to each reading as a present exchange between you and God. Focus on a word, phrase, or image that speaks to you, as you do in Lectio Divina. (Chapter 17) Chew on it, wrestle with it, ponder its relevance in your life. Listen to each story in terms of *relationships*. Which relationships are life-giving? Which are demeaning? Consider the stories about the use and abuse of power. How does this speak to our world today? What does God reveal about the way to love? About how to forgive? Notice, in the scriptures, the repeated assurance of the steadfastness of God's love for us through the ages.

LITURGY OF THE EUCHARIST

Sunday after Sunday, at churches all over the world, Catholics (and others) file up to the front of the church to receive the bread (host) and the wine. Watching this communion procession is like viewing a parade of humanity – the young and the old, the poor, the rich, the devout and the casual, male and female, the sick and the healthy. I always feel extremely privileged to witness this microcosm of the world. Even when communicants seem to approach the table on auto-pilot, or when the presider drones the words, "The Body of Christ" over and over, poker-faced, I find something deeply compelling about the ritual. What is it that brings this diverse group together – a group that may have little in common with one another except for this: Each, in her or his own way, is filled with a longing for something they cannot name. All are drawn to and fed from the same source – the source of all life. For the suffering and the sick, who more and more feel left out of the mainstream of life, being a part of this communion procession of human longing is validating and assuring.

The word "communion," broken down into its roots, reads: *at one with*. This "oneness" points to the God within all of us, and to our often un-nameable desire for this God. Therefore receiving communion is not a private "Jesus and me" encounter, but an opportunity to experience the God who dwells within one and all. Another way to refer to this oneness, this communion, is *The Eucharist*. "Eucharist" is a Greek word that means thanksgiving, or to give thanks to God. As we approach God's table we look through eyes of faith to give thanks for what God has done for us in the past, what God's doing for us in the present, and for what God will do for us in our tomorrows.

During the Eucharist we're called to remember, not as a past event, *but as a present experience*, the death and resurrection of Jesus Christ. I always say, "To remember is to experience anew." The very word, *re-member,* suggests embodiment. In the mystery of the Eucharist, we *re-member* our Lord in the breaking of the bread.

The total sacrificial giving of God's love in his dying and rising is present to all, in every generation. God's love is embodied in the bread and wine – taken, blessed, broken, and shared. We're called to open our hearts to God's unconditional love, mercy, forgiveness, and healing as we receive the intimacy of God's love in our communion. In turn, God asks us to love, forgive, and heal one another as we have been loved, forgiven, and healed. Our Eucharist strengthens us so we can reveal to the world the very face of God as evidenced by how we love one another. This is why I often ask my congregation to approach the Lord's table in a loving stance, to "carry" someone else with them to the table of the Lord, so that the intimacy received touches the person you carry as well. We become the embodiment *(re-member-ment)* of God to transform the lives of others.

Perhaps the most inspiring interpretation of the Eucharist for those facing an impending death is that of a heavenly banquet. Think of a generational meal shared with all those gone before us in faith. We call this the communion of saints - those who have passed, who are one with God, are *re-membered* and present at our Eucharistic celebration. So when we receive the intimacy of God's love at communion, we also receive the intimacy of *their* love.

The good news is...God calls us to this banquet every time the communion table is set. There we partake in the intimate love of God *and* of all those who have died. For the suffering, the sick, and the dying, and for those they will leave behind, the Heavenly Banquet offers such a message of hope and ongoing *communion* (being at one with) that includes past, present, and future generations.

EMPTY, FILL, AND SPILL - DYING AND RISING

To fully appreciate the Eucharist, it's helpful to participate through the lens of "Empty, Fill, and Spill." Deb and her husband Jerry, who was suffering from a serious heart condition complicated by diabetes, understood this. Despite the effort it took to get Jerry in the car with his oxygen tank, to stow the wheelchair, nail a parking space near the handicap ramp, and get themselves and their paraphernalia inside, coming to mass was a way for them to empty themselves of the frustration, resentments, and exhaustion that plagued them both during the week. It was a relief for them to come together to free themselves *of themselves*, to fill that space with the grace and power of

God's love and mercy, and to be sent out at the end of mass, renewed and refreshed, ready to face another week of spilling themselves out for the other.

Empty, fill, and spill is another way of experiencing dying and rising – the very essence of the Paschal Mystery. Through the reading of the Word and in the Breaking of the Bread Deb and Jerry, through Jesus's example, were encouraged to love out of their suffering. They filled themselves with God's love, forgiveness, and mercy, so that they could pass some of that along in the week ahead.

EUCHARIST FOR THE JOURNEY OF THE SOUL

Receiving the Eucharist is a timeless act of faith that nourishes us, in the span of a moment, across the entire Journey of the Soul (Chapter 1). For, in God, time is not linear but eternal. Moses speaks of this in Psalm 90:4: *"A thousand years in your eyes are merely a yesterday."* By sharing in this sacred meal God provides us with sustenance across all three phases of living. It is an invitation and an offering from God that asks the question once again, *"Will you let me love you?"* Through this meal God revives and restores us. Listen to God's loving invitation to us, in Isaiah 55:1-3:

All you who are thirsty, come to the water!
You who have no money,
Come, receive grain and eat;
Come, without paying and without cost,
Drink wine and milk!
Why spend your money for what is not bread;
Your wages for what fails to satisfy?
Heed me, and you shall eat well,
You shall delight in rich fare.
Come to me heedfully,
Listen, that you may have life.

I tell people, "Stop starving yourselves." Avoiding the Lord's table can become a kind of spiritual anorexia. Listen to the deep longing within. Say yes to God's gracious summons! Come to the table, eat, be filled and sustained by God's love. Only when you're filled can you begin to participate more fully in the expansiveness of God's love by extending that love to others.

SENDING FORTH

The Catholic Eucharist ends with the congregation being sent forth "to love and serve the Lord and one another." In other words, to spill the unconditional love, mercy, healing, and forgiveness out into the world. Our worship is empowering in this way, particularly for those facing a serious or terminal illness. For Amelia, for Deb and Jerry, for Rocco (whom we met at the beginning of this book) participating in an active and mindful way opened their hearts to a deeper, more mature faith. They'd leave, fortified to go out and face another week, confident that God's strength would sustain them as they extended God's love to others. As they were transformed, their faith, hope, and love, in turn, began to transform others.

Whatever your religion, and whatever the state of your health, consider opening yourself to the sacred rituals of your faith tradition. Together with individual spiritual practice, participating in communal worship can sustain and fortify you. If you're receptive to God's generative thrust, the love you experience in communal worship will flow into the world in a transformative way. Like a pebble tossed into a pond, love's gentle ripples will expand in all directions.

CHAPTER 19

The Expansiveness of Love

IN THE LAST months of my father's life he was confined to a nursing home. I walked into his room to find him seated in the chair beside his bed, his head hanging, eyes closed. He looked up and said to me, "Tommy, why am I here? I have nothing left! I love my house, my garden. Now I'm laying here in this nursing home. I used to walk, grow my roses. Now they have to hoist me from the bed to the chair. I can't eat, I can't see to read. Can't follow the racing sheets or bet on the horses. I can't even wipe my own ass. I'm useless!"

I said to him, "Dad, I can understand how you feel – a lot has been taken from you – but not everything."

"What have I got left? " he barked. "You tell me!"

I answered, "Your willingness to love."

He dismissed the notion with a wave of his hand. For my father, love was what you could do for someone - preparing a meal, cutting them flowers, perhaps passing along a magazine article or newspaper clipping. When my mother was dying she'd sit by the window and gaze outside. My father tended rose bushes for her, bringing her a daily bouquet. He planted a butterfly bush beneath the window and placed a bird feeder nearby. The last months of her life were spent enjoying the beauty of nature – a tangible expression of not only God's affection, but of her husband's love.

But now my father's repertoire for loving had been seriously curtailed, exacerbated by feelings of anger, resentment, and frustration.

His diminished ability to *do* the things he used to do made him feel powerless to love. But was he?

ALL THE WAYS TO LOVE

In the broadest sense, we can define love as the act of giving time, energy, and resources to another. In our culture, love usually conjures up ideas of romance, commitment, and reciprocity between two people. Romantic love and sexual attraction is often referred to as **eros**. This "falling in love" is characterized by infatuation and passion. The reason we "fall" into this kind of love is that it tends to just happen, driven by "chemistry" and fueled by desire.

Sometimes *eros* evolves into **familial love**, in which family members are tied together by bonds of affection, responsibility, and shared history. Familial love involves a strong sense of commitment, and demands tolerance, forgiveness, and gifts of time, energy, and resources. *Familial love* is evident between spouses or committed couples, parents and children, siblings and extended family.

Another kind of love shared between close friends is called **philia**. This platonic love is often nurtured through shared experiences, interests, and attitudes. It involves some validating commonality and is pursued and deepened by choice.

In all three instances (*eros, familial, philial*) love can, over time, become mired in practical dependencies and a sense of obligation. Our human tendency is to continually weigh what we're "getting out of it" and respond in kind. We can become scorekeepers in love, demanding and critical when our needs and wants aren't being met.

The highest form of love that can be extended to lovers, family members, friends and strangers alike is called **agape**. This is an intentional disposition, a conscious commitment to always look for the good of the other, consistently extending oneself in kindness and charity to everyone in our paths, regardless of whether they accept or reject it. Agape is also known as unconditional love. It is sacrificial, extended to all with no expectation of return. This is the love Jesus refers to when he says, "Love your enemies. Do good to those who hate you." It is at the heart of Christian teaching.

The Levels of Love

The highest levels of love, from 6 – 10, represent the movement toward unconditional love and are rooted in the spirit self. Levels 1 – 5 represent the more common forms of human or conditional love and are rooted in the ego self. Notice that levels 1-5 all come with expectations of return – a "quid pro quo" relationship. Transformative love (levels 6-10) is always given with no expectations of return or reciprocity.

10. I will choose to love you even if you are mistreating* me, even if you hate me, and even if you're my enemy.
9. I will choose to love you even if I'm experiencing physical, mental, emotional or spiritual suffering.
8. I will choose to love you with the permission to reject or accept my love.
7. I will choose to love you even if I don't like you or feel connected to you.
6. I will choose to love you generously and sacrificially with no expectation of return.

5. I will love you sacrificially with expectations of return.
4. I will love you generously with expectations of return.
3. I will love you minimally with expectations of return.
2. I will love you because I like you and feel connected to you.
1. I will love you out of a sense of obligation.

* It's important to note that when Jesus asks us to "love those who mistreat us," he's not asking us to be victims. Often, love requires setting boundaries that protect both parties, and these boundaries can produce the impetus for help that might otherwise be ignored. In fact, in cases of abuse, setting clear boundaries is the most loving thing to do and it is in the best interest of both parties.

Weighing these levels of love allows us to reflect on how much of the love we demonstrate to others is steeped in self-interest. It can also gauge the extent to which we allow God's unconditional love to flow through us to all those we encounter. Levels 1-5 are largely propelled by self-interest. When we love on those levels, we love and forgive *conditionally*. Levels 6-10 contain incrementally more of God and less of self, resulting in a love that is more pure, sacrificial, and transformative. When we love on these levels, we love and forgive unconditionally.

Our level of loving will always be commensurate with our image and experience of God. The more open we are to God's unconditional love, mercy, and forgiveness, the freer we'll be to extend that love, mercy and forgiveness to others. And, conversely, the higher our level of loving, the better we'll come to know God.

Given our human weakness, the challenges our culture places on us, and the limits of our faith, we simply cannot extend *agape* on our own. Instead we must surrender, admit that we aren't in control, that we're physically, emotionally, and often spiritually bankrupt. ***And only then, when surrender takes place, can we can transform our earthen vessel into a channel for divine love itself.*** This is the reason why the love shared during the dying process is so powerful - by opening ourselves to God's love and letting it pour forth, we share a sacrificial act that is the most vulnerable, most powerful, purest love of all – a love that comes *directly* from God and seeks nothing in return. Opening oneself to becoming a vehicle for *agape* not only graces each recipient, but it fortifies our own faith, blessing the journey we're destined to take.

MY DAD'S CHALLENGE - AGAPE

So, back to my dad...I've often said that love is an action, not a feeling. But "Big T" (as he was affectionately called) felt he couldn't act. He was becoming a prisoner in his own body. On the Path of Suffering most people experience this. As their world shrinks they become more and more self-absorbed. How is it possible, practically, to get out of your own way and love under those conditions?

I sat down and said, "Dad, throughout each day here you have opportunities to love." He shook his head and looked down. "You know what the first movement of love is? " I persisted. "A smile. When the nurse comes in to give you your pills you can smile at her. Ask her how her day is going."

Big T shrugged.

"You can do that, can't you? " I pressed.

He nodded. "I do that."

Warming to the prospects I went on, to drive my point. "And when the nurse comes to get you tucked in and settled, what are you going to do? "

"I don't like her," Big T snapped. "She wraps me too tight." His fingers inadvertently clawed the blanket covering his lap.

"Well then, even better," I replied. "She's giving you the opportunity to live the Gospel – to love at a higher level. To get outside yourself." It wasn't about "being nice." It was about communion. Oneness.

This solidarity of heart is achieved only by dying to self in the interest of others. The by-products of *agape* are steadfast inner peace and deep joy that are so much more life-giving than the fleeting flashes of optimism and happiness that are dependent on external conditions. Those who empty themselves in love experience joyful hope in God's consolation regardless of their physical condition, their prognosis, and even the ill will of others. They become peacemakers and bridge builders, empowered by God's spirit.

My dad spent the last month of his life extending himself as often as he could to his caregivers, his visitors, and his family. Words were difficult, as they had never been his strong suit, but by gesture and touch, a note written to his grandchildren, and eventually some simple words of endearment, he spent himself in love as best he could.

THE EPIPHANY OF LOVE

All of this hearkens back to Viktor Frankl's revelation during his march into the concentration camp, to St. Theresa's ability to love throughout her painful battle with tuberculosis, and to Eben Alexander's near-death experience. All captured the heart of the Gospel - the take-away point to live by and to die by. It has nothing to do with the Catechism or theology. It isn't an intellectual understanding of Christian thought and teaching.

What they discovered is much simpler, and at the same time much more challenging: in surrendering to the tragedy they faced, they saw clearly that *we are all asked to love as we have been loved by our God.* Loving unconditionally in *every* situation is our greatest calling – that our ability to love is what our lives are really all about. We were created through love, by love, and ultimately, for love. God wired us that way. The whole idea of resurrection is an outgrowth of love. Our search for meaning ends there – the meaning of life is to love unconditionally, despite our fate, our circumstances, or our prognosis.

In fact, love is the *only* thing that cannot be taken away. When a person experiences the loss of every earthly thing – health, the ability to play, to work, to think, to speak, when possessions, homes, jobs, professions, accomplishments fall aside, only love lives on. St. Paul said, in 1Corinthians 13:8, *"Love never fails."* By learning to expand our loving throughout the process of sickness and dying all of us can experience incredible empowerment and freedom. This kind of sacrificial love trumps everything else – it surpasses the sense of loss, outlasts pain, overrides anxiety. In fact, the Gospel of John says: *There is no fear in love, but perfect love drives out fear.* (1John 4:18)

HOW DO WE BEGIN?

Living in this way requires a new disposition, one that nurtures an internal climate conducive to sharing the kind of love that contains less of ourselves and more of God. This disposition includes four familiar yet essential components – *awareness, intention, practice,* and *consent.*

Awareness is the entre – awareness of the power of love, of our desire to love, of our natural inclination toward loving connections with others. Once the stuff of life begins to fall away, and we find ourselves in a transformative moment, our awareness is heightened. There is so much less clutter to muddle through. As Frankl, Therese, and Alexander had their eyes opened, so can we. The preciousness of a sunrise, the twinkle in the eye of a friend, the gentleness in the touch of a loved one – as the complications of life are stripped away, we become more aware of these essential gifts – and of God's hand in them. We begin to recognize that there is nothing of value except our ability to give love and our willingness to receive it. Not the love so often tainted with need and desire, love that during the green times is often entangled with dependency, but a purer, more selfless love - love given generously and freely with no expectation of return, with permission for others to accept or reject it.

Once we experience an inkling of awareness we can begin to embrace and cultivate an *intention* to reach out to others in love, to become the vehicle for God's love that is at the center of all that is. Without intention, awareness alone is just awareness. We can choose to act on it, or not. Intention sets the dynamic in motion, readies the heart, brings the necessary paradoxical union of surrender and desire that opens the floodgates allowing God's love to flow. It might begin as a mere droplet, then a trickle. And, given our human weakness, we might let a little through and then dam the waters once again. The wounds of the heart and any un-forgiveness that we carry are the stones that block the flow of love. This is why praying to God for healing and grace is a necessary component of our intention. Learning to let go and love is a recursive process, an ebb and flow. We might pull back, but it doesn't matter. Once we know we're connected to God, we know where we're going, then the when and how doesn't matter much. It's the intention and desire that count. This movement from awareness to intention brings about a momentum that holds a great deal of power and potential. The following quote attributed to 18th century German painter and novelist Johann Wolfgang von Goethe powerfully expresses this:

"The moment one definitely commits oneself, then Providence moves too. All sorts of things occur to help one that would never otherwise have occurred. A whole stream of events issues from the decision, raising in one's favor all manner of unforeseen incidents and meetings and material assistance, which no man could have dreamed would have come his way. Whatever you can do, or dream you can do, begin it. Boldness has genius, power, and magic in it. Begin it now."

Awareness and intention. The empowerment of loving. Perhaps the first glimmers of hope in the face of death.

As we get caught up in the vortex of the awareness of and intention to share God's love we're moved to **practice** and **consent**. Fueled by awareness and intention you'll begin to see tiny opportunities to reach outside yourself, to choose a loving stance rather than a reactive posture. This outward movement is liberating, because when we're extending ourselves to others, as we're noticing them, thanking them, listening to them, and sharing with them, our focus moves *away from the self*. It draws us out of ruminating about the past and grieving over the future. It shifts our obsessive thoughts about our treatment and possible outcomes to the person standing right before us. In fact, the act of loving places us squarely in the present. The fulcrum is tipped away from control and weighted instead with loving freedom. Though we might be in the process of dying, staying radically in the present means that in the given moment we are still *fully alive*. Our own pain and suffering take a back seat, if only for a moment or two. Giving up the self creates an internal space of consent that allows more of God into the mix. The transformation toward becoming who we are in God, (our true, spirit self) continues.

THE SACRED SPIRAL

Though we begin slowly, in small ways, this process has the potential to expand exponentially. Think of a spiral of ever-widening circles, with God (perfect unconditional and sacrificial love) at the epicenter. All of the energy emanates from that sacred center radiating across time and space. When juxtaposed over the linear timeline of life and death as we typically image it, the sacred spiral continues expanding, breaking down the barriers of here and beyond, its energy pulling us toward love like a whirlpool, while the ripples of that love expand outward. As our love spirals out into the world, we're also drawn inward where we recognize, perhaps for the first time, our true identity (the self we are in God's eyes).

Each intentional outward reach produces an equal inner movement. If, as the revelations of Victor Frankl, Therese, Eben Alexander, and others suggest, the approach to life and death portrayed by Jesus ring true, if we believe that God and love are one and the same, that God dwells at the core of our being and at the center of all that is, then we can begin to see love as our destiny.

No matter where we find ourselves on that evolutionary spiral, we can begin to let go and allow the natural movement toward deeper, purer loving to take place. True, Jesus and many of the saints and martyrs allowed the current of love to carry them to more highly evolved levels than we might expect to experience. But that doesn't matter. The beautiful thing about the spiral is that we start where we are, and no matter where that may be we're still connected to God and all that is. Some may realize the higher levels of love on this side of the grave. For others, it might take place on the other side. Either way, our destiny, our highest calling, is to become a vehicle for perfect love.

With a disposition honed through spiritual practices and worship we can begin taking small steps from acceptance toward transformation – by doing little things with great love.

Transformation of Self: – Relying on God's Love

I am the true vine, and my Father is the vine grower.
He takes away every branch in me that does not bear fruit,
and every one that does he prunes so that it bears more fruit.
You are already pruned because of the word that I spoke to you.
Remain in me, as I remain in you.
Just as a branch cannot bear fruit on its own
unless it remains on the vine, so neither can you unless you
remain in me.
I am the vine, you are the branches.
Whoever remains in me and I in him will bear much fruit,
because without me you can do nothing.

--JOHN 15

When we rely primarily on the God within, our ability to love unconditionally increases and the ego self diminishes. Heavy on unconditional love, light on conditional love (See below.)

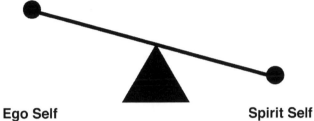

Ego Self

(Who I am in myself)

Spirit Self

(Who I am in God)

Evidenced by:

Need to Control --Willingness to Surrender

Trust in Self--Trust in God

Instinctive, protective reactions----------------------------Intentional loving responses

Holding on---Handing over to God

Unforgiveness---Unconditional Forgiveness

Many attachments---------------------------------------Sense of detachment

Self-Aggrandizement--Humility

Sympathy--Empathy and compassion

Defending self-interest------------------------------------Promoting interests of others

Feeling separate from all that is----------------------------Feeling part of all that is

Loneliness---Solitude and solidarity

Conditional optimism-------------------------------------Hope

Trying to manipulate God---------------------------Seeing God as loving and merciful

Staying on the surface of life----------------------------Embracing mysteries of life

Resistance to change------------------------------------Openness to change

Denial, resignation, acceptance--------------------------Transformation

Dependence on my strength----------------------------- Dependence on God's strength

Fear and anxiety--Inner stillness and peace

Self-absorption---Freedom from self

Glorifying Man--Glorifying God

Conditional love--Unconditional Love

Clinging to your False Self--------------------------------Accepting your True Self

CHAPTER 20

Doing Little Things with Great Love
(Expanding The Fertile Field of Your Heart)

MOVING TOWARD TRANSFORMATION OF SELF – TILLING THE SOIL

WHEN I TELL people that the first movement toward unconditional love is a smile, they often think I'm being cute, or trite. Simplistic and cheery. Or they think I'm overly sentimental, reiterating the words of an old-fashioned love song or a sappy old movie.

Before you dismiss my advice to smile often, consider this: Saint Teresa of Calcutta continually spoke of the value of a smile as a powerful vehicle for love and compassion. She has said:

- "Let us always meet each other with a smile, for the smile is the beginning of love."
- "Smile at each other. Smile at your wife, smile at your husband, smile at your children, smile at each other - it doesn't matter who it is - and that will help to grow in greater love for each other."
- "Every time you smile at someone, it is an action of love, a gift to that person, a beautiful thing."

In the face of great suffering, Saint Teresa sent her sisters out into the streets of Calcutta with these instructions. When powered by God's love, a smile, an act of selfless kindness, is a potent thing. A warm climate is created by the openness of a smile, and it is only in a warm environment that real sharing and understanding can be nurtured. Chronic, serious, or terminal illness can be isolating. As your world shrinks it's easy to feel lonely, and loneliness can kick up fear and anxiety. But a smile roots you in the present, beckoning others in.

So, extend yourself with the invitation of a smile and begin the process of "tilling the soil," turning over the hard-packed ground of our souls, impermeable from years of resistance and defensiveness. A smile...the first movement of love.

KATHY'S STORY

Kathy's older brother and I were childhood friends, and I remember watching Kathy grow from the little sister into a vivacious, outgoing woman. When she was diagnosed Kathy was married with two young adult children, a son and a daughter. She was an incredible fighter – taking her treatment in stride, always relying on her faith to fuel a positive outlook that convinced nearly everyone that she'd ultimately beat it. In fact, just several months before she died, Kathy walked a marathon on behalf of cancer research, providing inspiration and hope for others with the disease.

When Kathy took a turn for the worse her sister-in-law called me. "Father Tom," she said. "We need you to come. Kathy doesn't have much time left." I hopped the train to Boston and brought Barbara with me. Kathy knew we were working on this book together and she joked about wanting to "make it into the manuscript."

Barbara was blown away when she met Kathy. "The first thing I noticed," Barbara said, "Were her eyes. Blue eyes that communicated warmth and welcome. And her smile – instead of feeling as though we were showing up to offer consolation, Kathy's very presence made us feel like honored guests. Her ankles were swollen, her arms painfully thin, the bone structure in her face seemed exaggerated from the obvious weight loss. Despite her brightly colored robe and matching turban, her short curly hair escaping beneath, she looked much older than her 58 years. Yet none of this could squelch the inner glow that emanated from her. She directed the conversation away from her illness, asking us questions about the book, about my writing life and publications, about our work together at the church. It was an experience of being fully seen and heard – Kathy had this gift of reaching beyond herself. Being in her presence felt like standing on holy ground." And it all started with a smile.

POSITIVE RELATIONAL BEHAVIORS

By continuing to embrace the dispositions needed for spiritual growth – awareness, consent, and intention, we can become much more positive in our relationships, despite our suffering. A smile can prime the pump to pour forth other positive relational behaviors that will water and expand the fertile patch within, and spill over into the lives of others. Here are some characteristics I've seen manifested in those open to it. When we engage in these behaviors while struggling or suffering, we become vehicles for God's love.

THESE BEHAVIORS INCLUDE:

- being totally present to those around us
- performing little acts of kindness
- validating the feelings of others
- showing tender affection in thoughts, words, deeds, and touch
- accepting, unconditionally, what others do for us
- expressing appreciation through word, touch, tokens of gratitude
- affirming others by acknowledging their goodness
- encouraging those around us
- freely doing whatever has been agreed upon
- giving generously and sacrificially
- showing gentle patience
- accepting others' shortcomings, recognizing the pain beneath it

Just as Barbara felt in Kathy's presence, the recipients of these positive relational behaviors are profoundly touched by something much greater than the person before them. We can sense the presence and power of God. The sacredness of the moment is palpable and unforgettable.

Here are a few additional examples of those on the Path of Suffering who discovered strength in weakness, light in darkness...

PHIL'S STORY

Phil (whom we heard about in Chapter 17) was married to Sandy for 33 years, and they enjoyed a rich, full life together. Phil was Catholic, Sandy, Protestant, and they regularly practiced their faith together.

To their disbelief, Phil was diagnosed with gall bladder cancer that had spread to the liver and in no time found himself in treatment at Sloan Kettering. Life had turned on a dime, and four months later Phil was spending what would be last days in a hospital bed, Sandy by his side.

Though Phil was grief-stricken, he made it a point to reach out to everyone in a spirit of love. As his nurses, doctors, and caregivers entered his room, Phil smiled, engaged them in conversation, inquired how their day was going, learned their names, asked after their families.

Phil was finally released from Sloan because there was nothing left to be done. As he was being rolled from his room on a stretcher to be transported home via ambulance, a crowd formed on the floor – doctors, nurses, janitors, food service staff and orderlies, all wishing him well. Embraces, warm words, tearful goodbyes.

When the ambulance arrived at Phil's house, the driver took Sandy aside, telling her about the crowd that had gathered. "Your husband must be a famous man – I've never seen that kind of a send-off."

The fact was, Phil had ministered to each and every one of them, reaching beyond his pain and loss. He became so much more than his illness, and, in fact, he had profoundly touched many lives, evangelizing by example. Here was a man who, with God's help, extended himself in love and care for others, with no expectation of return. Phil died a week later. His witness has provided his wife and all those who cared for him with a legacy that continues to give them great hope. And each day it began with a smile.

Phil had, in many ways, tilled the fertile field of God's boundless love. He was able to access the living and loving presence of God that was within the field of his heart during his final ordeal, harvesting the fruits of the spiritual work he'd done throughout the years. Sandy shared that Phil gave her a gift in his dying. It was a silver lining in a tragic moment.

FROM A SMILE TO POSITIVE RELATIONAL BEHAVIORS

Mother Teresa and her Sisters of Charity, Kathy, and Phil were able to get out of their own way (through God's power) and extend themselves to others in love, in spite of difficult, challenging circumstances, in the midst of loss and great sadness. If we think about the fulcrum, each of them tipped the scales toward unconditional love, and shared the freedom and joy that comes with it. In emptying themselves they became channels through which God's unlimited love could pour forth. The reason the recipients of this love were so deeply moved is that this love is the purest love of all – because it flows from the very heart of God.

Doing little things with great love, transforming the ordinary into something extraordinary, is really only possible one day at a time, one encounter at a time, each approached with great humility, acknowledging our human weakness and absolute inability to love out of our suffering on our own steam. This is what Jesus talks about when he tells us we must be like little children, totally dependent on and grateful for the spirit that's so much larger than our will and ability. Every hour of every day will require a continuous handing over, a willingness to fail, and a recommitment to begin again. As theologian, philosopher, and mystic Meister Eckhart has said, "Be willing to be a beginner every morning." As we become more dependent on God and less on self we grow in confidence in the promises God has made to us, as we see God's strength manifested in our day-to-day living. This process becomes a testament to God's love and fidelity, more powerful than words, or even prayers. When both the patient and caregiver become dependent on and open to the working of God as their source of strength they can transform a loving partnership into something much deeper. They can become "soul partners" – not only cooperating together in administering the patient's care, but lovingly pointing the other toward the face of God.

This kind of loving dependency is not only a powerful consolation, but it builds a deeper faith and trust in God to carry us forward toward the greater relational work we're called to do in our sickness and dying. And it's possible for it all to begin with something as simple as a smile.

"Not all of us can do great things. But we can do small things with great love."

— SAINT TERESA OF CALCUTTA

CHAPTER 21

Forgiveness and Healing

A NUMBER OF years ago I led a pilgrimage to France which included an excursion to Lourdes. For one of our pilgrims, a faithful parishioner named Gary, this was the reason for the trip. Suffering from terminal cancer, the visit to Lourdes offered him great hope. We walked among hundreds of pilgrims, many in wheelchairs pushed by their nurses, and sensed something quietly electric in the air. The level of faith and devotion was palpable – or perhaps it was hope. Our group visited the grotto where the Blessed Mother appeared and walked the Stations of the Cross set in the rocky hillside. A number of us waited with scores of others for the privilege of being bathed in the healing waters. We proceeded in a line leading into a canopied cabana, where multi-national volunteers helped us discretely disrobe and draped us in white, towel-like shrouds. The baths, fed by the mountain stream, are set behind a curtain. As your turn approaches you can hear the quiet sounds of others being immersed – the murmur of voices, a gentle splash and a gasp (the water is cold!). Each pilgrim enters alone. The atmosphere is one of sacred mystery, much like a baptism.

Gary was profoundly moved by the experience. Directly afterward he went off by himself to try and discern the seismic shift inside him. He believed that he'd been healed, that his cancer was gone.

That night Gary had a vivid dream about his boyhood. His father had been an abusive alcoholic and young Gary had had to constantly defend his mother. As a result he was often battered and beaten. In the dream his father appeared to him, not as an inebriated bully but as a new creation - reaching out to his son with gentleness and love. It was a dream of forgiveness, healing and reconciliation, a vision that freed Gary from the burden of bitterness and resentment that he hadn't realized he'd been carrying.

Gary's cancer persisted and soon afterward he died. But the real healing was what had taken place *inside*. He was strong, brave, and loving right up until the day he died. Gary died happy, free, unencumbered, and unafraid. In the process he'd shown others how to live and how to die with grace. But, it wasn't Gary's strength that brought about this transformation. It was his willingness to be open to God's working in his life. Gary's story is an example of how seasoned faith, forgiveness, and healing become conduits for God's love – and the keys to a joyful death.

WHERE IS THE LOURDES IN OUR LIVES?
Most of us won't go off to Lourdes. We likely won't have a transformative experience like Gary's, waking up from a dream healed and whole. For most of us the work of forgiveness is exactly that – hard work. In the "field" of our souls, the act of forgiveness can be thought of as removing the stones from the soil. Back-breaking toil, but an absolute necessity if we hope to be able to plant the seeds for an abundant harvest.

If the thought of grappling with forgiveness feels like more than you have the strength to deal with, consider this – lugging the emotional baggage of a lifetime is even more taxing, and much more difficult on the final leg of life's journey.

When their father died, twin brothers Michael and Joe inherited the family lumber business where they'd both worked side-by-side for years. Joe had ambitious ideas about how to expand the business. Michael, the more hands-on of the two, preferred to work the yard, talking to contractors and building relationships with a handshake. He left the financial decisions to Joe. Joe convinced his brother that they should borrow some money to buy out a competitor and corner the local market. Michael reluctantly agreed.

Soon afterwards a large national hardware chain moved into town. Ultimately the family business failed and both brothers were left holding a hefty bank loan. Michael never forgave Joe for "forcing" them into debt.

Thirty years later, when Michael was dying of prostate cancer he continued to rail against his brother, ruminating on how his life might have been different, how he and his wife could have had the money to get the place in Florida they always wanted, how his daughters could have gone to better schools, and how it was all because of Joe. Michael's wife tried to convince him to let it go, to reconcile with his brother. They'd had a good life, despite the loss of the business. She arranged for Joe to come by to visit, to mend fences, but Michael refused to see him. Michael died a bitter old man, when he could have rewritten the story of his life by revising the final chapter. Doing so doesn't erase what happened before. It just changes the ending.

How Difficult it is to Forgive

Forgiveness has been defined as *"an intentional and voluntary process by which a victim undergoes a change in feelings and attitudes regarding an offense, lets go of negative emotions such as vengefulness; with an increased ability to wish the offender well."*

There are many health benefits associated with forgiveness. Studies have shown a correlation between forgiveness and lowered blood pressure, reduced levels of stress hormones in the blood, a boost in the immune system, and a reduction in common complaints such as back pain, headaches, and digestion problems. If this is the case, why is forgiveness so difficult? Theologian and author C.S. Lewis has said, "Everyone says forgiveness is a lovely idea, until they have something to forgive ..."

Our culture sends us mixed messages about forgiveness. On the one hand, many of us pay lip service to the value of forgiving those who hurt us. But the media sends a very different message: for every offense, there's a price to be exacted. This plays into our natural instinct of self-preservation, survival, and security. When we realize that what's happened cannot be undone, society tells us that we can at least regain a sense of control by striking back. The retaliatory response may be swift and automatic or careful and calculated. We see it in the number of lawsuits that bog down our court systems. It plays out just as powerfully in our homes, schools, and neighborhoods.

We feel justified in these retaliatory behaviors because we believe it's our right – maybe even our responsibility - to even the scales. The downside is that the need to get our pound of flesh holds us prisoner.

Once we feel the other has paid dearly enough, we might inch toward a kind of **qualified or conditional forgiveness.** But because the emotions of both have been bruised and inflamed, all it takes is the *suggestion* of a slight and the cycle begins all over again. Over time, if the hurt hasn't been healed, this ingrained vengefulness can harden into hatred. We perpetuate the hurt by transmitting it to others and can't help but begin to see ourselves through a negative lens. This destructive self-labeling is often reinforced as we unconsciously act out of our pain, damaging relationships and continuing the dynamic.

Sometimes the natural inclination to fight back is curbed by a sense of propriety or pride. We might find out-and-out vengefulness distasteful. Perhaps we don't want others to see us as vindictive. Instead, we get our revenge indirectly. We become masterful at the art of nonverbal messages, using our expressions as weapons of disdain or disregard. Even if the person apologizes, it can be difficult to accept, because we're so blinded by our own hurt. We might grudgingly offer some level of forgiveness, while waiting for any and every opportunity to disparage the other. When the person who hurt us is faced with some misfortune there may be a moment when we allow ourselves to think, *Ha! He had it coming!*

An alternative message society sends is that when you're hurt you should just somehow let it go, or toughen up in order to overcome the emotional damage through sheer will. Some respond by withdrawing from the one who caused the pain. Others turn the pain inward, or deny their pain by repressing or denying it, or rationalizing it by making excuses for the perpetrator. We all know someone like Carolyn – it was common knowledge that her husband had had a string of affairs. While obvious to everyone else, Carolyn seemed to have selective blindness. It was easier for her to deny the pain than to deal with the realities of it. Similarly, Elaine's adult son David had, for the most part, cut his mother out of his life. Elaine rationalized his behavior, explaining, "David has such a big job! It's impossible for him to leave the city. And then there are all the business trips..."

While aggressive and passive responses may seem very different, they're all rooted in *control*. If we're focused on control we cannot be present to love anyone or anything. Remember the emotional physics of the fulcrum – when we're heavy on control, we're light on love.

OUR PERSONAL PAIN

Time and time again, when I talk to people about forgiving those who hurt them, I hear the same response: "But Father, you have no idea what he/she did to me..."

Everyone's pain, the injustice or betrayal they've suffered, feels so uniquely and individually dehumanizing. When we suffer hurt at the hands of another, especially someone we call family or friend, it's hard to believe that anyone can understand the depth or breadth of that anguish. We feel that this particular sin against us is the justifiable exception to Jesus' command to forgive seven times seventy times.

But this experience is universal, a hallmark of what it means to be human. Regardless of the seriousness of the wound, we all go through the same struggle to forgive. However, contrary to what our feelings dictate, the process of forgiveness is *not* impossible.

I often tell the story of Rwandan Genocide survivor Immaculée Ilibagiza who survived for 91 days hidden with seven other women in a tiny 3x4 foot bathroom of a local pastor's home. From inside they heard the Hutu rebels hunting down and viciously murdering their Tutsi neighbors, friends, and family. Immaculée's father, mother, two brothers and countless members of her extended family were brutally slaughtered and thrown into shallow graves. In her book, *Left to Tell – Discovering God Amidst the Rwandan Holocaust*, Immaculée describes her difficult journey to forgiveness and peace – a process wrought with setbacks, doubts, and negative emotions. She recognized early on that the only way she could possibly forgive was through the unconditional love and healing power of God.

Immaculée went through all of the typical stages - naming and getting in touch with the hurt, dealing with the resulting powerful, negative feelings. Due to the horrendous nature of the crimes, the instinct to retaliate was nearly overwhelming. She prayed consistently and fervently, not denying her feelings, but acknowledging that she was powerless over them:

> "Please open my heart, Lord, and show me how to forgive. I'm not strong enough to squash my hatred – they wronged us all so much... My hatred is so heavy that it could crush me. Touch my heart Lord and show me how to forgive."

Immaculée opened her heart to forgiveness, but as she moved through the process she realized that the intention and the practical reality were two different things. When the Rwandan conflict came to an end and Immaculée revisited the scene of her family's murders she realized that forgiveness was more than a feeling and an intention – it was all about letting go of the desire to retaliate. She writes:

> "I went straight to bed when we arrived at the camp without talking to anyone. My soul was at war with itself. I'd struggled so hard to forgive but now I felt duped for having done so: I had no clemency left in me. Seeing my home in ruins and visiting the lonely, forgotten graves of my loved ones had choked the life out of my forgiving spirit."

As in any hurtful situation, the pain can resurface. It usually requires us to relinquish it over and over, to ask God for the grace not to strike back. Immaculée turned to God still again:

227

"Forgive my evil thoughts, God," I prayed. "Please...as you always have, take away this pain from me and cleanse my heart. Fill me with the power of your love and forgiveness. Those who did these horrible things are still Your children, so let me help them, and help me to forgive them. Oh, God, help me to love them." A sudden rush of air flooded my lungs. I heaved a heavy sigh of relief, and my head dropped back on the pillow. I was at peace again. Yes, I was sad—deeply sad—but my sadness felt good. I let it embrace me and found that it was clean, with no tinge of bitterness or hatred. I missed my family desperately, but the anger that had gripped me like a returning malignancy was gone. I also prayed for compassion as well, I asked God for the forgiveness that would end the cycle of hatred—hatred that was always dangerously close to the surface."

We might have a tendency to dismiss Immaculée as a saintly exception, especially in light of the often petty unforgiveness we hold on to. We feel the same way about Jesus hanging on the cross, asking his Father to forgive his executioners. It seems super-human, impossible. It would be, if forgiveness were dependent on *us*. But it isn't – *it's dependent on God.*

EXPERIENCING GOD'S UNCONDITIONAL FORGIVENESS

My parishioners have heard me say, thousands of times, "You can't carry unforgiveness." Unforgiveness is more damaging than any disease - a barrier to God's love that makes it impossible for us to freely experience the love others attempt to extend to us.

There's a "mantra" we recite at every Catholic Christian liturgy – *Lord, have Mercy...Christ have mercy...Lord have mercy.* It isn't about Catholic guilt, or groveling before God. It's about acknowledging the universal need for God's grace, forgiveness, and healing. It's about being mindful of the way our own remorse and regret over the mistakes we've made and the hurt we've caused weigh us and others down and be vulnerable enough to stand honestly before God as a sinner. Developing a healthy sense of humility, and acknowledging our *own* need to be forgiven is a prerequisite to being able to forgive another. We first have to experience God's unconditional forgiveness. We can't give to others what we don't have.

The church has a beautiful sacrament called "Reconciliation" (sometimes called Confession) to help us enter the mystery of God's mercy for us. When Catholics go to Confession, the priest is the embodiment of God's merciful love. When done well, the priest will help you experience God's compassion and mercy. The stones that weigh you down are removed. I watch people enter the confessional wrought with worry and regret, and leave with a sense of renewal and freedom. My job isn't to forgive them – God has already forgiven them, offered the gift of mercy in the very instant that they sinned. My job is to help them unwrap the gift freely given. I always send them forth with this directive... "Now go out and forgive as you've been forgiven."

A PROCESS FOR FORGIVING OTHERS

There are a number of steps that are helpful once we've decided to begin the worthwhile work of extending forgiveness. Forgiveness isn't a skill to be mastered – it's a disposition and practice empowered by our willingness to surrender our hurts and to take a leap of faith. All of it is rooted in God's power, not ours. The following process illustrates some of the ways we can best cooperate with God's spirit, and open ourselves in faith.

- **Name the Hurts**

We must begin by clearly naming our hurts. We all carry a combination of conscious, subconscious, and unconscious hurts. I think of them as scratches, cuts, or ruptures. Uncovering and acknowledging these hurts is critical – we can't heal wounds we're unaware of or unwilling to see. For some it's helpful to talk it through with a trusted friend or family member, not for the purpose of pointing blame, justifying our reactions, or looking for "solutions". The very process of choosing the words to best describe the hurt can help clarify these feelings. Another approach is to journal, recording the hurtful incident on paper. There's a natural tendency to paint ourselves blameless and the other as the sole perpetrator. While this is sometimes the case, part of the process of naming the hurt involves accepting responsibility for whatever role we may have played in the dynamic, whether intended or not.

• **Suspend the Impulse to Retaliate**

While reflecting on your pain you conjure up the feelings anew, in effect exposing yourself to the injury all over again. This can trigger the impulse to retaliate, to defend yourself, to strike back either passively or aggressively. To wish the perpetrator harm. Here is where a leap of faith is required – and the willingness to be real with your God. Don't deny any vengeful or negative thoughts; instead, articulate them to God, admitting that you're powerless over them, acknowledging that it is only through God's power and mercy that you can relinquish them. Prayers don't need to be complicated – you can get right to the point: *God, every time I think of the way he hurt me I just want to lash out at him again. I want him to feel the same pain that I do. Help me let go of this, because I just can't do it on my own...*

As anyone in AA will tell you, admitting your powerlessness is the first step toward recovery. The humility of surrender prepares a space for God to enter. Repeat your prayer as often as you need to, every time the negative, vengeful thoughts creep up on you. Letting go is a process and a practice. It takes time.

Strive to see the person who hurt you through God's eyes. Open yourself to accept that this perpetrator of hurt also has a story, and that what he or she did to you was a result of this. If not healed, hurts are always transmitted. Ask God to help you see through a lens of compassion.

This is a recursive process, full of stops and starts. Through compassion you glimpse the heart of the other and then are ambushed again by the pain of the injustice done to you. Let go, begin again, asking God for the grace you need.

• **Begin to Experience God's Healing Power**

The only way we can forgive is to treat the wounds that drive our impulse to retaliate. All wounds require attention and care if they're ever going to heal. Imagine a gash on your hand. Left untreated it will fester and become infected, affecting your overall health. Emotional wounds are no different.

I suggest a simple symbolic ritual. Imagine God's love and mercy as a healing balm. Place your hurt in your hand and name it. Then, apply the healing balm, massaging your hand as you pray: *Father, I believe you are healing this hurt. I do not doubt it. Thank you for your healing love.*

Barbara found this prayer difficult, because the childhood wounds she suffered were so pervasive – in fact they seemed to have greater power over her than did her faith. I'd encourage her to pray anyway and she'd complain, "How can I tell God that I believe and do not doubt when I *do* doubt? "

Faith always requires the art of surrender, the suspension of disbelief. Reluctantly, with doubt always pressing in, she continued the process. She was impatient, and every time she saw evidence of the wound surfacing again – an over-reaction to some hurt, the way that being disregarded pushed all her buttons – she'd tell me that it wasn't working. And I'd say, "Be faithful to the process."

How do you know if healing's taking place? Day to day, you're likely not to notice the subtle changes. But after a month or two of applying the healing balm you may notice some of the signs of inner healing:

- less self-talk and focus on the past, less time ruminating on the hurt
- emotional hot-spots cool down – you respond more than react
- a growing awareness of God's compassionate mercy toward you

- a greater willingness to accept responsibility for your part in the dynamic
- you begin to recognize the hurt that drove the other
- you become freer to love in all situations
- a greater willingness to invite God into the ever-deepening process of examining the more mysterious wounds of life
- feel a pull to deepen your faith and witness to the working of God in your life
- consider initiating the process of reconciliation

Every time Barbara would complain to me that it just wasn't working, I'd ask her, "Are you freer now to love than you were before? Are you more compassionate toward others who are struggling? Can you recognize the wounds that caused your family to hurt you? " Her answer was always "yes..."

Will you backslide sometimes? Of course. But it's important to remember that healing takes time, and the signs of inner healing are gradual and subtle. Look for the fruits and freedom of healing. And remain faithful to the process.

As the process continues, you begin to see through the lens of compassion and understanding. You practice taking a leap of faith, asking God to heal your pain. Your intention is to surrender the hurt, relying on God's strength rather than your own, acknowledging how difficult it is, recommitting to the process every time you backslide.

- **Pray for the Good of the Other**

The next step is to begin the practice of praying for the person who hurt you. In Luke 6:28 Jesus says: *Bless those who curse you, pray for those who mistreat you.* Perhaps the very idea is unpalatable. If that's the case, admit it. Begin your prayer honestly: *Lord, I'm having trouble being sincere about this, but help me to pray for _____, for her good, for her healing. Help me to see her as you do.* Or, simply acknowledge that God loves that person: *Lord, I lift up_____to you. Thank you for loving her.* Your intention will begin to change your heart, and with each passing day your prayer will begin to feel more sincere.

• The Possibility of Reconciliation

Making a decision to try to reconcile with the other is a choice we have to make. It's not always possible and sometimes not desirable. Depending on the nature of the hurt, setting healthy boundaries may be the best thing for everyone involved. But reconciliation can be a blessing if we're aware of the fact that the relationship cannot possibly go back to the way it was before. Again, I think of Jesus talking about the impossibility of pouring new wine into old wineskins. What was, is no more. If you expect that reconciling will restore the relationship to what it was prior to the rift, you'll be disappointed. You've both been changed by the reality of what took place. When attempting to re-establish a bond it's important to understand that you're creating something different and new. A more seasoned relationship.

If you do reconcile, you have to be prepared to redefine the connection between you both. As in any new relationship, it will take time to test the waters, to negotiate your roles, to discover who this new person is and how you will best relate to one another. If you're trying to reconcile with someone who hurt you, it might be best not to begin with, "I forgive you for what you did…" The fact is, from the other's point of view, the scenario might have looked very different. Instead, you might begin with, "I realize the situation was complicated. We both made mistakes. I'm asking you to forgive me for whatever role I played in it. If I hurt you in any way, please forgive me. And I forgive you as well." In this way your move to forgive cannot be interpreted as an implied "holier-than-thou" judgment. Acknowledging the complexity of the dynamic and assuming responsibility for your role lessens any defensiveness the other might be feeling.

You also have to face the possibility that you may reach out to reconcile and the other may refuse. Carla and her sister Lisa had been estranged for ten years. When Carla got sick she began the process of forgiveness and decided it was time to try and reconcile with her sister. She called Lisa, explained that all was forgiven, that she missed her, and that she hoped they could talk. Lisa hung up on her. The rejection Carla felt kicked up many of the old feelings of anger and resentment. Her wound was torn open and she had to begin the process all over again. She learned that forgiveness and reconciliation do not always go hand in hand, and that forgiveness needs to be unconditional, a gift given with no expectation of return. Whenever you initiate a reconciliation, it's important to go in accepting whatever response you might receive - another leap of faith. As I always say, "Love never imposes."

FINAL REFLECTIONS ON FORGIVENESS

The challenge and value of forgiveness has been contemplated by many great minds. Reflect on the following quotes as you consider how forgiveness may heal some of the wounds of the past and fill your tomorrows with peace.

"An eye for an eye only ends up making the whole world blind." – Mahatma Gandhi

"We must develop and maintain the capacity to forgive. He who is devoid of the power to forgive is devoid of the power to love...Forgiveness does not mean ignoring what has been done or putting a false label on an evil act. It means, rather, that the evil act no longer remains as a barrier to the relationship. Forgiveness is a catalyst creating the atmosphere necessary for a fresh start and a new beginning. It is the lifting of a burden or the canceling of a debt. There is some good in the worst of us and some evil in the best of us. When we discover this, we are less prone to hate our enemies."

– MARTIN LUTHER KING, JR.

Moving toward forgiveness involves looking at the complexity of difficult situations – those of your own life and those of others - through eyes of compassion. Things that happened in the past can be revisited and reflected on through the broader, gentler perspective that often evolves and crystalizes during the sobering experience of facing an impending death. In the next chapter we'll explore the questions to ask that can free us to forgive, help us embrace our vulnerability and losses, and open the door for the loving conversations that can transform us and those we love.

CHAPTER 22

— ⌒ —

Story Telling – Healing the Wounds of Your Life
(Expanding the Fertile Field of Your Heart)

I HEAR A lot of confessions.

Every Saturday afternoon, parishioners line the ends of the pews, waiting their turn to come and unburden themselves as best they can. During Lent, besides Saturdays, we have confessions every Tuesday evening. Once a year, my associate and I have a <u>Day of Reconciliation</u> that starts at 9am and goes non-stop until 11pm. I've been doing this for 16 years, and I don't leave the confessional until the last person is finished. Last year I didn't lock up the church until 12:30 am. People carry in their lists of shortcomings – times they hurt themselves or others, occasions when they couldn't muster up the love they should have demonstrated. The simple day-to-day stuff – angry words, impatience, little white lies that gradually add up then weigh you down like pebbles in your pocket.

And then there are the heavier stones – retaliation and revenge, sins of omission, the fruits of addiction, betrayal, jealousy, lust, adultery. I listen. Nothing much surprises me because the "small stuff" and the "big stuff" are all driven by the same engine – and that engine is a person's *story*. My response is always the same: "Let's talk about it – what's the hurt that's driving the behavior? And what's the story that's caused the hurt?" After nearly half a century of confessions and as many counseling sessions, here's what I can tell you for certain – everybody, I mean *everybody*, has a story.

The problem is, sometimes we become hardened by our own stories. The hurt may have been so ongoing that the routine of it became the norm of our lives. Others may have told us to stop being so sensitive, to toughen up, to deal with whatever hand we've been dealt. In order to save face we push away the hurt and "get on with life." Cover our vulnerability and keep the story buried in the deepest parts of our souls.

Others take the opposite approach, telling the story over and over again, fanning the flame of anger and righteous indignation in a cathartic manner. Either way - denying the story or by making it a perpetual negative refrain, the wound never has the opportunity to heal. Instead, the stones of hurt and the resulting sin begin to multiply, blocking God's fertile patch within.

We also have a tendency to feel isolated and diminished by the hurtful stories of our lives. We see others as "having it all together," as people who surely came from "better", less dysfunctional families, well-adjusted people clearly deserving of more satisfying relationships, who have been respected and treated accordingly. We fail to see beneath the veneer and to understand that every member of the human family carries his or her own portion of hurt. And that these hurts, instead of serving to separate us, can actually become a bond that unites us in compassion.

Conversely, some of us look at others who are struggling and feel a bit smug and self-satisfied. *Thank goodness we're not like them. Why can't they just get it together? If they'd only do A, B, or C...* This kind of thinking can be a red flag – if we easily jump to judgment or are indifferent to the struggles of others, it may mean that we haven't really gotten in touch with our *own* stories. Compassion is the byproduct of gentle realism, of accepting the brokenness of human life, including our own.

Think about the conversations in your life that have really mattered, in which you and another laid all your cards on the table. When you exposed your vulnerability and shared your personal truth – and in doing so, revealed to yourself things you hadn't fully understood before. Maybe a handful of times during our lives we're able to turn ourselves inside out to another, and in doing so are able to better understand and embrace who we are.

As our lives are winding down, nothing is as satisfying as a loving conversation in which the stories of a lifetime are shared. Revisiting these stories in the context of a waning life can put many things in perspective. If you've done the work suggested in the previous chapters, looking back over the stories and situations that have defined you can help make meaning of the life you've lived. It can illustrate all the ways that your presence in this world *mattered*. Sharing these stories can be a gift to those you love, allowing them to get to know you in a more intimate way than they ever had before. You might think that you don't have a lot to tell. But I'd say, from experience, never underestimate the power of your own story or that of someone you love. There's always more to it than meets the eye.

WHY IT'S IMPORTANT TO TELL OUR STORIES

In my parish, we've placed the following adage on the front page of our bulletin: *See a face, learn a name, hear a story, and love one another.* Reflecting on and then telling our stories through a lens of gentle realism is so helpful as we journey through life – and never more important than during the final stages. Most of us tend to look at our lives as a series of fragmented pieces, rather than holistically. When this happens, it's natural, consciously or unconsciously, to assign greater significance to some stories and to live out of these stories. We forget that we are really the sum of the parts. In the case of a dominant negative story, it can often overshadow legitimately good memories. The negativity becomes a lens through which we see ourselves and the world. A dominant negative story can hold us back and limit our life choices.

Barbara has spent a good deal of time grappling with her story. The adult child of an alcoholic, she grew up knowing her parents loved her. But her father's alcoholism controlled the family dynamic. As the years passed, his addiction worsened and eventually killed him. He was only 49 years old.

Barbara's extended family and friends knew little of the escalating struggle going on behind the closed doors of her home. Her father never missed a day of work, rarely drank outside the house. Her parents' relationship was dominated by her father's drinking – he would get drunk and her mother would yell and scream at him, while continuing to enable his addiction. All of this caused Barbara to become invisible to both of them. As an only child there was no one with whom to process any of it. In fact, the craziness eventually became the norm. As a child and then a teenager she denied the situation to the point that not a single one of her friends suspected.

By the time she began college Barbara had become an over-achiever, taking 21 credits a semester and earning a place as one of the top ten scholars in her freshman class with a 3.98 grade point average. On the surface, everything was fine. She continued to excel, to become an accomplished musician, author, mother, and teacher. Except, as time went on, the need to be perfect, to distinguish herself, became a source of constant stress and anxiety. It wasn't until she was 40 years old, after having committed herself to some serious spiritual and emotional work, that she was able to recognize the ways in which she'd been unknowingly living out of her story. Taking a backseat to the turmoil of an alcoholic household, she was often inadvertently disregarded. The fact that the alcoholism was kept a careful secret made her feel as though she had something shameful to hide. Over-achieving was a way to say, "Do you see me now?" It also served to compensate for the deep-seated sense of being part of a family with a "shameful" secret. The implications of this story produced a "hot button" in her life – in any situation in which she felt overlooked or ignored Barbara would respond disproportionately, demanding to be heard, sharply and adamantly articulating her point. Those on the receiving end wound up paying the price for the hurt caused by her family story.

The reason to get in touch with your story is not to point a finger or blame another for the choices you've made or the direction life has taken.

If your life has been dominated by a negative event, the redemptive part of embracing a story is to begin to acknowledge the complexity of it, to come to terms with the fact that another's pain affects everyone, and that we all transmit pain that hasn't been brought forward for healing. By examining your story you can begin to transform your wounds into *sacred wounds* and become a compassionate wounded healer. Nothing is more fulfilling during the process of sickness and dying than being able to use your wounds and redemptive suffering to better understand, empathize with, and heal the lives of others.

The forgiveness and healing discussed in the last chapter now needs to be brought home, applied to all the tender places inside that we defend and hide. This process removes the stones of hurt and rocks of resentment that litter the fertile field of our souls.

WE ARE PARADOXICAL PEOPLE

Telling your story truthfully, with a sense of gentle realism, involves perceiving, and embracing *paradox*. "Paradox" occurs in situations that seem to be steeped in contradiction. Something appears to be one way, we think we have a handle on it, but then some aspect of it doesn't fit into the neat category to which we've assigned it. Openness to paradox allows the understanding and acceptance of the human condition as "both/and" (both a saint and a sinner) rather than "either/or" (either saint or sinner). In sharing our stories, we need to begin to accept the complex totality of who we are. Over-identifying with one side or the other is a distortion and a denial. And as we begin to recognize this in ourselves we also begin to understand that *everyone* is a living, breathing paradox.

This was powerfully illustrated when my sister Maureen presented me with a beautifully framed plaque. When she'd spotted it in the gift shop she immediately thought of me. It was a poem that captured the parts of myself I was proud of, as well as those I was not so proud of - the "me" I put out there and the "me" I sometimes try to hide.

240

<u>What Shall I Say About the Irish?</u>

The utterly impractical, never predictable,
Sometimes irascible, quite inexplicable, Irish.
Strange blend of shyness, pride and conceit and
Stubborn refusal to bow in defeat.
He's spoiling and ready to argue and fight,
Yet the smile of a child fills his soul with delight.
His eyes are the quickest to well up with tears,
Yet his strength is the strongest to banish your fears.
His hate is as fierce as his devotion in grand,
And there is no middle ground on which he will stand.
He's wild and he's gentle, he's good and he's bad,
He's proud and he's humble, he's happy and sad.
He's in love with the ocean, the earth and the skies.
He's enamored with beauty wherever it lies.
He's victor and victim, a star and a clod,
But mostly he's Irish in love with his God.

---Source Unknown

The truth in this paradoxical poem resonated powerfully in me. I truly am neither this, nor that. I am both/and. And, in so many ways, so are you. This is what it means to embrace *all* aspects of our stories and understand that they are part and parcel of who we are. This is the holistic reality of you that God loves.

HOW TO BEGIN TELLING OUR STORIES

Before finding an empathetic ear, it's important to do a bit of soul-searching. You need to gently probe your primal responses, blow the dust off of memories, some long buried. What you discover can be extremely revealing, and possibly downright revelatory.

To help you in this story search, I'm asking you to take some serious time to consider the survey questions that follow. A first step would be to invite God into the process. Ask the Holy Spirit to lead you through the questions and into the mysterious synergy of memory, emotions, and truth. Try to flesh out your answers with examples or anecdotes. Your responses will reveal the patchwork of your life – the joys and sorrows, celebrations and regrets, triumphs and losses. Responding honestly to these questions can help uncover wounds that need healing as well as blessings to acknowledge and celebrate.

Be on the lookout for the following as you contemplate each question: If a specific incident or repeated scenario comes to mind, consider the way it impacted you. How did you respond to it? Looking back, was your response reasonable or exaggerated? Did you express your feelings or repress them? Perhaps you denied the emotions altogether – in other words, you refused to acknowledge the anger or hurt. If this was the case, as these questions poke at your past you might experience a crack in your armor that allows you to look at the complexity of the situation for the first time.

Keep in mind that there are emotional and behavioral clues that point to capped feelings. Over-reacting to the experiences of others, displaying a disproportionately intense response when someone offends or disagrees with you, reacting to stressful situations by either running away (avoidance) or by aggressively confronting them. If you have an overwhelming need to control, a difficult time accepting affirmation or affection, or follow the "one strike and you're out" rule – meaning that it's hard to forgive or to trust anyone who's hurt you – these kinds of responses often signal a buried hurt that has been dominating your inner world. If you find yourself, after still another uncomfortably familiar confrontation, asking, "How did this escalate to this level?" chances are you're being bullied by your "shadow self," by past hurts that need to be healed.

Addressing these questions honestly is not a process to accomplish in a single sitting. You might want to create a journal where you write down your responses. Come back to the questions that puzzle you. Sleep on them. *The questions you find the most difficult are likely the ones that deserve the most attention – they have the most to divulge.* This is an ongoing process that requires a serious commitment, so stick with it! As you elaborate on your answers, be sure to include words like: *because, although, except, but, however, since, still, yet, on the other hand –* these are the qualifiers that help clarify and nuance your story, suggesting the reasons, motivations, contradictions that point to layers of truth. Begin to examine the story of your life through a larger lens. The goal isn't to tell these stories as a journalist would. Instead of focusing on the mind, allow your heart and soul to temper your responses. Don't look at your story as good or bad. Try not to judge. Tell the story in order to let go, to celebrate, to wonder, to forgive – in other words, to accept the whole of it as part of the mystery that is you.

If you delve into the process with the mindset that you're being led by God, what is revealed can be considered sacred – set apart for God. Think of God as the compassionate listener who will never judge or condemn you. Our all-knowing and all-loving God will not be surprised by any aspect of your story, will not assign blame or inspire guilt. You might begin by reflecting on Psalm 139:

> *Lord, you have probed me, you know me:*
> *you know when I sit and stand,*
> *you understand my thoughts from afar.*
> *My travels and my rest you mark;*
> *with all my ways you are familiar.*
> *Even before a word is on my tongue,*
> *LORD, you know it all.*
> *Behind and before you encircle me*
> *and rest your hand upon me.*
> *Such knowledge is beyond me,*
> *far too lofty for me to reach.*

God can temper your responses, and provide a level of loving objectivity. As you view your role in these stories you'll see yourself and others as both hero and fool, victim and oppressor, and realize, perhaps for the first time, that this is truly the nature of humanity. Looking through the broader lens of God helps us humanize others who have affected our lives in negative ways. Realizing that they, too, have stories makes it so much more difficult to dismiss them as no-good, unreliable, irresponsible, or insensitive. To recognize that if they were to answer these questions, they would have complex stories to tell that ultimately drove their behavior. That they're as vulnerable as we are, and that God looks at them with compassion as well.

If you're still having difficulty believing that God is a compassionate God, it might be because the father figure in your life was overly strict, demanding, critical, punitive, distant, or even absent. Because our culture images God as a paternal figure, we often inadvertently project onto God the qualities we've come to know in our own fathers. If you find that this is true, your prayer might be, *"Help me Lord, to see you as you are – to recognize your love and compassion for me. Season my faith so I might know you in new ways."*

THE QUESTIONS OF YOUR LIFE

As you consider the questions that follow, we encourage you to apply them to the various stages of your life. **How would you answer in regard to your childhood, adolescence, young adulthood, middle age, etc.?** You'll see that your answers may change based on your life at each stage, and the way your answers are altered through the years is worth looking at. Try using a notebook to write down your thoughts in regard to these questions. You can divide each page into columns, one column for each life stage to make it easy to see the evolution over time and the cause and effect nature of changing relationships.

Sharing your responses openly with another is a powerful way to begin the healing process. Work your way through them, a couple at a time. Then go back and revisit them from time to time, digging a little deeper, being a little more open and honest, embracing what was with freedom and a sense of generosity.

FAMILY:

1. Describe your relationship with your father.
2. Describe your relationship with your mother.
3. Describe your parents' relationship.
4. Describe your relationships with your siblings.
5. Describe your relationship with your spouse and children.
6. How did you celebrate as a family?
7. How has your family dealt with suffering, chronic illness, dying, or death? How did this impact you?

FRIENDS, MENTORS, INFLUENCES:

1. Who do you care about the most? Why?
2. Who has affirmed you the most and perceived you in the best possible light?
3. Which have been your most life-giving relationships? Describe the ways these relationships were positive for you.
4. Which friendship(s) do you value most and why?
5. Who has had the greatest influence in your life? Why and how?
6. What are you passionate about? What moves you? Why?
7. What have been the high points of your life? Describe them.
8. What are your greatest accomplishments? How were you able to accomplish them?

STRENGTHS AND CHALLENGES:

1. Tell about a time you overcame a difficulty. How did you accomplish this?
2. What qualities do you see as your strengths?
3. What has been your most challenging relationship and why?
4. What angers you? Is it the result of a life event, and if so, what?
5. What are you most afraid of losing? Why?
6. What is your greatest regret? How might you have responded differently?
7. When did you feel the most misunderstood and why?
8. When was the time you felt most betrayed? How did it happen?
9. Tell about a time you let someone down. How and why?
10. Tell about a time you failed. How and why?
11. What has been your biggest disappointment? Why?
12. What has been your greatest loss? What contributed to this loss?
13. What qualities do you see as your weaknesses?
14. What have been your biggest challenges? Why?
15. What "pushes your buttons" and makes you respond with disproportionate intensity? How might the disproportionate response relate to a particular life event?
16. How do other's perceptions about you differ from who you really are? What is the reason for this discrepancy?

SPIRITUAL JOURNEY:

1. Who has encouraged your spiritual growth and development?
2. Describe the times you were most aware of God's working in your life.
3. In what spiritual practices have you actively engaged?

4. What do you think is the meaning and purpose of your life?
5. In looking back at both the highest and lowest points, where do you see the hand of God?

TELLING YOUR STORY TO ANOTHER

After channeling the questions through the compassionate acceptance of God, it's time to reach out to another and share your story. Telling your story is different than pondering your story. The very act of selecting the right words, and then actually verbalizing them empowers you to actually *hear* your story. You process it using different parts of the brain, like taking in a story via audiobook, versus in print.

The process of talking about your story with a friend or an objective third party can be extremely validating. It can be like shining a light into a dark corner. Articulating it aloud diffuses some of the power the story has over you. But it also opens you up to greater vulnerability, as family members or friends can never be as open and accepting as God. And sometimes, when discussing with a spouse, lover, or family member, filters can go up, or their responses may challenge your perceptions.

But, this too, is important. To begin to understand that others in your life may see the same situation through a very different lens can be enlightening. Barbara compared this dynamic to writing a novel. When fleshing out the cast of characters it's critical for the novelist to step into the shoes of each character, to know their backgrounds, life experiences, and motivations, all of which color their individual points of view. Every action and reaction has to be crafted through the emotional landscape of each particular character. This is what generates the most important elements in successful fiction: tension and conflict. While tension and conflict are what drives a book that's hard to put down, in real life, the effect is very different. Instead, we might begin to argue or withdraw, to rush to judgment, resentment or un-forgiveness.

Of course, there is no need to divulge everything to everyone. It can be helpful to examine the various aspects of self in the context of story-telling. Consider the following:

- The **public self** can be defined as how others see you.
- The **private self** is the 'you' that very few see.
- The **hidden self** is the part of you that you don't share with any-one, though you're aware of it.
- The **unconscious self** is the part of you that is *not* seen by even you, and is revealed only through symbols, dreams, and creative expression.

It's helpful to ask whether there's a large gap between your public and private selves. How much do you keep private, and what informs this distinction for you? How does this affect your relationships? How much of your hidden self might be driving negative or hurtful behaviors? Can you see a cause and effect connection between the two?

Part of the process of storytelling as loving conversation is to rec-oncile the various aspects of the self so that the gap between the pub-lic, private, and hidden selves can assimilate into a cohesive whole, thus eliminating discrepancies that do not serve you well. Should you choose to gently reveal parts of your private or hidden self to another, you might enable them to better understand what makes you tick. You give them the opportunity to become more empathetic and compassionate toward you, and this dance of vulnerability and trust can deepen the relation-ship. On the other hand, if the person you choose to reveal these private and hidden details to hasn't grappled with their own shadow self, you open yourself up to judgment and criticism. So, choose wisely.

It's never advisable to rush to the deepest, most complex parts of your story. A gradual unfolding is important, beginning on common ground. Moving from the familiar, or agreed upon aspects of your shared history, and then wading into deeper water. Staying in the first person point of view (in other words, using *"I"* statements: *I remember... To me it seemed...The way I recall it...From my point of view...It made me feel...*

*At that point in my life I believed...*is important. These observations are so much easier for another to accept than *"you"* statements (*You hurt me when...*) or declarative judgments about other people or situations: *He was mean and selfish... She never liked me...* The "I" statements show your vulnerability, and in doing so, encourage your listening partner to open up in kind. The depth and openness you bring to your story is commensurate with what you're able to take in from another. The opposite is also true – another can only understand your story to the extent to which they've unearthed their own. That said, sharing honestly can become the impetus for your listener to begin the same exploratory process. The dynamics of your story might resonate with parallels in their own lives. In this way you can become the leaven that can raise their "bread of life."

Often, the hardest part of broaching the stories of our lives with others is knowing how to begin. If you're at all uncomfortable, you can use this book as the jumping-off point. You might start by saying, "You know, this book I've been reading encouraged me to take stock of my life by looking at a whole series of questions." (You might show your partner the list.) "I took my time answering. It was hard, but I learned a lot. I realized there were a lot of stories I've never told. I'd like to tell you a couple. Hearing them might even open your eyes to a few of your own stories..."

Then, tell your story gently. Don't look for a particular response from your listener. If he or she challenges or disagrees with you, simply accept that. Instead of engaging in an argument your response might be, *"Interesting how differently we see it."* Then let it go.

CRAFTING YOUR "STORY ENDING"

The most powerful part of discovering the various threads of stories that wove the tapestry of your life is that it isn't over until it's over. To go back to Barbara's analogy to novel writing, what makes a book memorable is the way the character grows and changes based on the events of the story. The most powerful characters have faced great conflicts, confronted challenging issues, and emerged from them more compassionate and resilient people. The way your story ends depends on you. You can choose to ruminate and hang on to past hurts, or to use them as a springboard to understanding, healing, and forgiveness. You can choose to highlight threads of bitterness or wisdom, resentment or compassion, defensiveness or forgiveness.

The rest of this book is intended for those who choose *love* as the ending to their story, who gather the multicolored threads of experience and tie them together in a tapestry of gratitude, forgiveness, and healing. All of the work you've done in the field of your heart – doing little things with great love, fasting from negativity, embracing forgiveness and healing – this prepares you for the road ahead. This legacy can become a gift for friends, family, and acquaintances to cherish. It is the ending that goes beyond acceptance and peace and extends to spending whatever you have left in love. And it is an ending enhanced by completing the rest of our earthly journey with the support of a *soul partner*.

For I am already being poured out like a libation, and the time of my departure is at hand. I have competed well; I have finished the race; I have kept the faith. From now on the crown of righteousness awaits me, which the Lord, the just judge, will award to me on that day, and not only to me, but to all who have longed for his appearance. – 2 Timothy 4:7-8

Transformation of Others

Relying on God's Love

In John 15:11-13 Jesus said to his disciples:

*I have told you this so that my joy might be in you
and your joy might be complete.
This is my commandment:
love one another as I love you.*

CHAPTER 23

Becoming a Soul Partner

WE'VE ALL HEARD lovers refer to the object of their affections as their "soul mate." Usually they're referring to someone with whom they experience a strong, immediate attraction. Soul mates feel as though they've known each other forever, that they were destined to be together.

A *soul partner* is different – a spouse, family member, caregiver, friend, or clergy person who helps you to recognize and access the working of God in your life and the lives of others. After both partners have experienced transformation, allowing God's unconditional love, forgiveness, and divine healing to change the fertile patch within them into a fertile field – they can enter into relationship with God and each other in more profound ways.

Soul partners share a new attentiveness and awareness of God's hand in not only their lives, but in the lives of all people. Because of this they have grateful hearts, using every opportunity to affirm God's work in the world, and to witness to the power of God in all lives. The Psalms of praise and thanksgiving resonate powerfully with them, and the psalmist's voice becomes their own. This charism and grace that soul partners experience can rouse a similar awareness in others, to help transform their life view, and serve as a compassionate audience for the stories of others. These spiritual companions provide a sharper lens through which we can begin to see the significance and meaning of our suffering. They can freely discuss the Journey of the Soul, as well as the Path of Suffering. Soul partners experience a communion, a oneness with God and the other, sharing a deep sense of intimacy. When either partner finds him or herself in the dark hole of despair, the other can offer hope. A soul partner lights the way of faith, keeping it always before their partner, during times when pain and suffering can cause them to forget.

How are some people able to achieve this kind of relationship? Only when both parties are living out of the spirit self do they have the potential to become Soul Partners. When every interaction is exchanged in and through the spirit self, *everything* is transformed. The entire experience becomes something sacred.

Caregiver ←——————→ **Patient**
Spirit self　　　　　　　**Spirit self**

In some cases, one partner is walking the Path of Suffering led primarily by the spirit self – the other may still be rooted in the ego self. Whenever the ego-self dominates, it generates negativity that can eventually wear the spirit-led partner down. In these cases the spirit-led partner (caregiver or patient) would benefit by finding a soul-partner elsewhere who can support them spiritually and prevent them from slipping back into a defensive, ego-based posture.

In thinking about a soul partner, consider the following spiritual practices that typify this spiritual relationship.

Soul Partners will:
- **Pray together**

Prayer takes many forms. Soul partners might recite formal prayers together, pray the rosary, offer intercessory prayers or speak directly to their God in the presence of the other. Perhaps they read a Psalm aloud, or a poem. There is a favorite prayer that I give to soul partners to pray together. It is known as the *Prayer of Abandonment* by Charles de Foucauld. It is a prayer of great hope in the power of surrender. Praying it primes the spirit for the release that may not yet feel comfortable. I ask people to pray it with faith, humility, and intention, whether or not they feel ready to own the words. Praying it with a soul partner, discussing your respective feelings, can be revealing. Questions of faith and doubt, fear and vulnerability, freedom and control are mined in the recitation of this prayer. Proclaiming it together can help us let go of our expectations and take small steps toward complete reliance on God.

Prayer of Abandonment

Father, I abandon myself into your hands; do with me what you will.
Whatever you may do, I thank you: I am ready for all, I accept all.
Let only your will be done in me, and in all your creatures –
I wish no more than this, O Lord.
Into your hands I commend my soul:
I offer it to you with all the love of my heart, for I love you, Lord,
And so need to give myself, to surrender myself into your hands without reserve,
and with boundless confidence, for you are my Father.

Some soul partners share prayer journals where they've written their most intimate thoughts about and responses to God. Dee and Denis (who we read about in Chapter 6) regularly used their journals as a way to share their journey of the soul.

Also, when one cannot pray due to illness or great suffering, the soul partner becomes the proxy, praying on their behalf. A powerful example of this comes from Jennifer. Jen is the lead cantor at our parish – bright, bubbly, vibrant, full of life. Married with three children and a nurse by profession, she was shocked when diagnosed with MS before her 40th birthday. At her lowest point, she found herself unable to pray, but being an engaged member of the church community, she had many others praying for her. Here is her reflection, shared with our community as a powerful witness:

"I am completely overwhelmed by the outpouring of love and light sent my way last night. The prayer/good thoughts sent out for me made an anxious moment become still and prayerful amidst the noise. Your thoughts became my shield and I am grateful. I am a true believer in prayer. But there are times when our hearts and even our souls may feel empty. As humans we give so much and sometimes we forget to fill our cup. I spoke about this a couple weeks ago at a women's gathering--about how community became my prayer when I simply couldn't pray. And community became my hands when I could not use them and my feet when I could not feel them. But the idea of 'You were my prayer when I did not have a prayer in my heart' is a concept so hard to articulate but I have been spirit-led to say that our voices begin as a single voice, but then become part of collective voices all praying and thinking about one person and they somehow become a single solitary voice...they blend together and gather such strength and power. I can see it and hear it right now and I wish you could too, because the words I am attempting to use are flat, and how I see it is so beautiful."

- **Engage in open, honest, loving conversations** about their personal image of God - their relationship with God, and the struggles and consolations they've each experienced on their respective journeys of faith. Story telling (Chapter 22) and loving conversations (Chapter 24) take on greater significance between soul partners, as the stories and events of one's life become more clearly rooted in God. Soul partners encourage forgiveness and healing, expressing not only empathy, but compassion. They affirm and validate the feelings of the other because they listen with merciful hearts. Soul partners explore and discuss the Journey of the Soul they both are taking, preparing one another for their indwelling.

- **Encourage each other to higher levels of loving**
Soul partners support and challenge one another to love unconditionally, to become vehicles for God's love as they're emptied by suffering. They remind and model for their partner ways to "do little things with great love." An example of this was when my dad told me how he didn't

like one of his nurses who wrapped him too tightly and I encouraged him to thank her, to relate to her, to respond to her kindly.

- **Feed each other the Word of God**

As you begin to read the Word of God to one another is it is important to keep in mind what St. John XXIII said about prayer: "Pure Prayer is listening to God, conversing with God, and being silent before God." As the ego self diminishes and the spirit self grows, the Gospels take on deeper meaning. Once the incessant self-interest begins to shrink, the soul is much more open to hear and experience God's word. You begin to have a deeper hunger for the Word of God which will sustain and strengthen you. Jesus reminds us again, *One does not live by bread alone, but by every word that comes forth from the mouth of God.* – Matthew 4:4

Passages that once seemed "throw-aways" suddenly come to life, ripe with insights.

- **Meditate together**

Sitting together in holy silence, with the intention of accessing God's presence within both of you, can be a peaceful and life-giving practice. Greater than words, steeped in mystery, the practice of surrender becomes a dress rehearsal for the great "letting go" inherent in death and in grief. I often think of my friend Kathy, whose mother was suffering from dementia. She and her mom often sat together in solitude, in a peaceful and loving communion, the presence of God palpable between them. This silent, sacred vigil pointed to another, deeper level of communication that was taking place. (See Chapter 17.)

- **Reverence the Cross**

At this point in the journey the Cross/Crucifix serves as a powerful symbol. In the past we might have reflected on the Cross of Christ as something totally other, as Jesus' destiny. Now we begin to also recognize it as our own. Soul partners understand and strive to embrace their respective crosses. They might meditate on the following scripture passage of

Jesus addressing his disciples: *"If anyone wishes to come after me, he must deny himself and take up his cross daily and follow me."* – Luke 9:23.

What always amazes me is that Jesus didn't just talk the talk – he walked the walk. Along the road to Calvary he walked with humility, dignity, and grace, loving in every interaction. He died to show us how to surrender the ego self to something greater. Soul partners reflect on the cross together, exploring its meaning and relevance. This reflection can be transformative. As Kathleen Dowling Singh says in her book, *The Grace in Dying: A Message of Hope, Comfort, and Spiritual Transformation*:

> "The symbol of a crucible is a great symbol for the transformative potential of suffering. The crucible---like the cross, the West's primary symbol of transformation---represents a situation in which one is held in place, to endure and experience what is. The crucible of suffering holds the whole being on the line of immediacy, committed to the experience of the present moment. And, on the line of immediacy, as Walt Whitman powerfully put it: "I and this mystery, here we stand."

This reminds me of Phil, who we met in Chapter 17, in the final stages of his disease, raising a glass and proclaiming, without bitterness or regret, "Here I am Lord...what can I say? "

Soul partners encourage one another to focus on loving rather than becoming obsessed with their own suffering - to reach out rather than turn inward where we can become self-absorbed with anxious thoughts, self-talk, recriminations, or any form of negativity that fuels the flames of mental, emotional, and spiritual suffering. This can only happen when we stay radically in the present moment – not going back to the past or racing toward the future. In a sense, we must become nailed to the cross of our own suffering, giving up all in order to allow the spirit self to emerge and dominate. Loving soul partners can help one another stay in that crux of a place, in seeming contradiction. It is in this paradoxical place that transformation occurs. Whenever I hear the following memorial acclamation proclaimed at mass – *Save us, Savior of the world, for by your cross and resurrection, you have set us free* – I understand that Jesus set out to free us, not from our suffering, but from *ourselves*.

- **Bless One Another**

After several debilitating strokes, Ray - a family man, husband, father and grandfather - found himself in a nursing home. He seemed a shadow of his former self, diminished in so many ways. He had run his own business, loved to summer on the Jersey shore with his kids and grandkids, and enjoyed traveling with his wife of over 50 years. Now he depended on others to get him in and out of bed. He needed to be fed and diapered. The prognosis was bleak.

Ray recognized that he was limited in many ways, but in spite of that (or perhaps because of it) certain other things that he'd never understood before became crystal clear. As he looked back over his life he began to see all of the ways God had worked in his life. He realized that this God of love had been with him all along. Ray's insight was a huge blessing to him – one he felt compelled to share with everyone who crossed his path – his wife and family, friends, visitors, caregivers.

Barbara visited him in the home, and as she said her goodbyes, Ray surprised her, motioning for her to come closer. She leaned over the bed, thinking he was going to whisper something in her ear. Instead, Ray reached up, took his thumb and made the sign of the cross on her forehead. Lips slightly parted, his eyes clouded with a distant look, as though seeing something Barbara didn't. Like Kathy, Ray had turned the tables, the consoled becoming the consoler. Barbara knew that, once again, she was standing in a sacred place.

Soul partners make it a point to bless one another. I encourage them to make the sign of the cross on one another's foreheads and say, "God bless you. May you see the working of God's love in your life." This opens the door to conversations about their awareness of what God is doing for them in their present lives. Another blessing I encourage, while signing the cross on a partner's forehead, is this, "God/Jesus loves you, and I love you too." This blessing is a reminder that they are the embodiment of God's love for the other.

- **Embody God's Love for the Other**

Soul partners become vulnerable enough with one another to allow themselves to be served and cared for by the other. They begin to see that the caring heart and hands of the soul partner are, in fact, God's heart and hands. They also recognize that the illness provides an opportunity for each of them to do what Jesus preached – visit the sick, feed the hungry, care for the dying. If both the one being served and the one who serves can see this, everything changes. There is no more bitterness or resistance on the part of the patient over feeling helpless, no more resentment on the part of the caregiver for the never-ending responsibilities. Both begin to see the practical aspects of day-to-day care as something sacred and holy. The patient provides the opportunity for the other to love in deeper ways, and together they embody the following scripture: *I was hungry and you gave me food, thirsty and you gave me drink, naked and you clothed me, sick and you cared for me, in prison and you visited me. – Matthew 25:35-36*

During the Holy Saturday service, I saw a man walking with great difficulty to the baptismal font to bless himself. After the service Linda, a parishioner, introduced Richard to me for the first time. He was struggling with the symptoms of ALS, and told me how difficult it had been. An engineer by trade, he was a man who liked doing things for himself. This became a challenge as the disease progressed – not being able to walk unassisted, or button his shirt. When his wife and daughter tried to help him, he'd become angry and resistant, creating tension and anxiety between them. Richard and I met in his home on many occasions. Over time, we became soul partners, sharing deep spiritual conversations, discussing where God was in this process. Richard was a man of deep faith, but he had a need to always be the one in control, to be the provider, the helper, the fixer in the household. On top of that, he was feeling an "absence of God." Before his illness he often "heard God's voice" but that voice seemingly vanished. After still another fight about Richard resisting his wife and daughter's care, I told him that what he was doing was pushing God away. Rejecting God's love, enfleshed, as offered through his family. This stopped him short. He just had never seen them that way. This revelation changed the dynamic in the family. He also came to appreciate, first-hand, God's love and presence for him in and through his family's care.

After Richard's death his daughter told me how the opportunity to care for him had been such a gift. As the ego self diminished, Richard became more himself, his true self revealed, the self that relished and cooperated with his family's care as a manifestation of God's love. And his family drank deeply of the joy of doing His will.

- **Receive Communion and the Sacrament of Anointing**

Soul partners will see that they experience the oneness inherent in the Eucharist. One may bring communion to the other in order to provide the "bread of heaven" or attend Eucharist together. This is a powerful form of nourishment for the soul. The care-giving partner can also arrange for the patient-partner to receive the Sacrament of the Sick – anointing with sacred oil, laying on of hands, and praying the prayer of faith for healing.

SOUL PARTNERS BOTH BENEFIT

As I continued to walk with Richard on the Journey of the Soul, we engaged in many of the preceding spiritual activities. I came to love his smile, and he eagerly awaited our conversations. We relished the gift of our soul partnership. Richard and I shared our fears, our faith, and, yes, even our doubts. His illness became the impetus for all of this.

After his funeral, Richard's wife and daughter took me out to dinner, and talked about the ways the journey had changed during the course of Richard's and my relationship, and how what had been viewed as tragedy had been transformed into an opportunity for deep faith. They presented me with a notecard that Richard had dictated to them for me before he died. It read:

Hi Father Tom,

There is nothing better in this world when two people open their hearts up to one another to discuss life's issues at hand. I've got to say, that I've really looked forward to all of our visits. Father, I don't believe this was a coincidence, I think the Holy Spirit put this one together. I've learned so many points which have been missing during my life. And for this I praise and thank God.

Love, Rich, Mary Jane, and Tina

The life-giving, honest, loving, reciprocal experience of becoming Soul Partners is possible between any people of mature faith, and even more powerfully realized if both partners have experienced suffering. We saw it between Dee and Denis, I've seen it between friends. I've seen it between people of vastly different ages and of different faith traditions. Richard taught me a lot about the way each partner benefits and grows in a transformative way. Most powerfully, soul partners recognize God in the other, and gently and consistently help the other remember that and live out of it. Together, they traverse life on a deeper level, seeing far beyond the very real challenges inherent in the dying process. They become each other's spiritual guides, encouraging the faith necessary for sacred surrender.

But, most of all, they help expand the pervasive myopic view that focuses on controlling the disease at the expense of everything else. They guide each other toward a bigger picture, a larger more miraculous story. Together they embrace mystery, in a sense of awe and wonder. They begin to see what most can't – that they are standing on holy ground – that they always have and always will.

CHAPTER 24

Opening the Door to Loving Conversations

IN LIFE, THERE'S a first and a last time for everything. Barbara often talks wistfully about her children, now adults, remembering the years when they were small. "Sometimes I feel saddened by the fact that there were so many 'last times' that I never recognized," she explains. "There was a last time I tucked them into bed, a last time I bathed them, a last time I held their hands crossing the street – and the preciousness of those moments was, in some way, lost on me at the time because there would always seem to be another opportunity. I just didn't realize how fast time moves along."

This becomes particularly sobering when we, or someone we love is slipping toward death. There will be many 'last times' in regard to all kinds of things, due to the constrictions of disease. But even more important than the shared activities we can no longer engage in are the thoughts and feelings we hold close to our hearts. The practical demands of physical care can sap so much energy that little is left for the emotional needs of both patient and caregiver, making meaningful conversation a challenge. It's so important to take advantage of our ability to express our inner musings to those we love before it's too late. When days are running out like sand in an hourglass, the number of words and sentiments we can share dwindles as well. There is a point at which conversation can become impossible due to the effects of the illness, the treatment, or medication. So, when terminally ill people are in what I call the "green zone" – when they're still mentally aware and articulate, I tell them it's time to have an intentional talk with everyone who really matters. Once they slip into the "yellow zone" where they mostly sleep, and might move in and out of consciousness, the chances of getting any meaningful words out dramatically decreases. And people sometimes suddenly enter the "red zone" where they'll lapse into unconsciousness. When that happens they've already experienced the "last time" for sharing words of gratitude, forgiveness, healing, and unconditional love. Therefore, planning loving conversations is critically important, and the sooner, the better.

WHY WE'RE AFRAID TO TALK ABOUT DEATH

There are a myriad of reasons why both loved ones/caregivers and the terminally ill have apprehensions about discussing death. If either party is in denial, of course, meaningful conversation is out of the question. However, even when both parties are complicit in their denial, their relationship will become mired by underlying stress that will express itself in all kinds of indirect and negative ways.

In my experience with the dying, they're often pretty clear about their fears around discussing their impending deaths. The most common reservation they express is that they don't want to distress family and friends. The sight of their loved one's grief and anxiety is more than they can bear. They don't want to feel responsible for a spouse's or child's emotional pain. Sometimes, when relationships are broken, or long-standing conflicts between family members exist, the prospect of introducing any additional strain feels devastating, and is therefore avoided.

Most people worry about becoming a burden to loved ones, and talking about the possibility feels like treading on thin ice. "I just don't want to go there," confided Sophia, who had been diagnosed with 4-5 years to live. "The thought of having someone wipe my behind – of losing my dignity, is just..." She shook her head, her eyes filling with tears. She waved her hand before her, as though she could sweep the subject away.

Other people facing death, confined to a hospital bed, find themselves in an environment that isn't conducive to discussion about difficult topics. At any given moment medical staff might appear to poke, prod, medicate, or otherwise intrude on an intimate sharing. No one wants to be interrupted in the middle of a life-and-death conversation.

At the end of life, long-held secrets, unfinished business, and unresolved conflicts tend to rise to the surface. Sometimes, in an attempt to keep these unpleasant memories buried, the person will shut down, afraid that discussing the past might open a floodgate. Or perhaps the dying person was never adept at articulating feelings, and contends that "you can't teach an old dog new tricks." As though breaking their life-long habit of "playing their cards close to the vest" is the equivalent of betraying who they've been.

In the case of a patient who's fought very hard, discussing death may represent "giving up." But as I always say, it's pretty hard to fight on two fronts. If you're fighting the disease right up to the end, there'll be no energy (or time) left for accomplishing the very real work of dying.

Sometimes even when the patient is anxious to talk, loved ones are resistant. When family members refuse to engage in conversation about an approaching death, it's often because they haven't yet faced or dealt with their own vulnerability, mortality, or losses. They're hit with the realization that if this can happen to someone near and dear, then it could also happen to them, or to anyone else they love. This can be overwhelming, and to keep their fear in check they refuse to discuss it.

Some, like parishioners Joe and Ellie, married 45 years, were like two peas in a pod. Neither wanted to imagine life without the other, and so they upheld a tacit agreement not to discuss Joe's terminal illness, each "protecting" the other. Another very different couple, Nick and Joyce, whose relationship of 35 years was characterized by turmoil around Nick's repeated infidelity, also struggled to discuss Joyce's diagnosis. Nick's guilt and shame over the past and his inability to express his remorse caused him to avoid any conversation besides the practicalities of his wife's treatment.

OVERCOMING FEAR AND RELUCTANCE

Remember, on some level, everyone involved in something as profound as death wants to discuss it, talk it through, deflate the huge taboo surrounding it. Explore it with someone they trust. Discover a safe place where they can be vulnerable, where they can face fears and anxieties or simply express what they're feeling inside. No one really wants to navigate this uncharted territory alone. Such conversations ideally occur between the patient and a beloved spouse, family member or friend, but it could also be with an objective third party – a clergy member, psychologist, or even a nurse or other caregiver. No matter how uncomfortable it might initially feel, or how reluctant a partner might be, there are ways to gently open the door to sensitive, caring conversation.

SETTING THE CLIMATE FOR CONVERSATION

Meaningful exchanges can only take place in a warm, accepting climate. I like to say that when we enter into relationship with another, an energy field is created that strives to keep us connected. I've named this energy field the "WE." Think of a Venn diagram – "WE" is the area in the middle made up of the cross-section of individual circles representing you and your partner. The "WE" is a powerful living dynamic between both parties that depends on relational energy in order to thrive. This shared relational space can be small (in the case of less intimate relationships), or in well-established, older and deeper relationships, it can grow to be quite large, the shared, intersecting section becoming even bigger than the individual pieces.

"WE" energy can be positive (the by-product of consistent affirmative inter-relational behaviors) or negative (which comes from destructive relational behaviors.) The "WE" is sustained by *both* the positive and the negative, always seeking to stay connected to an energy source. Engaging in positive energy is usually intentional, while putting out negative energy is automatic – think of it as the default setting. If there's little deliberate positive energy working within the "WE," the negative energy automatically kicks in. We've all witnessed this - married couples that fight constantly, but stay together year after year. One or the other will pick an argument they've had a million times before that nobody wins. Friends and relatives marvel at the way they return to this dynamic over and over again. When you think about it, it makes perfect sense – negative energy is preferable to no energy at all. Without energy (negative or positive) the relationship (The "WE") will die.

This dynamic is never as apparent as when walking the Path of Suffering. The caregiver totally spends him or herself – perhaps bathing and dressing the patient, managing meals and medications, assisting in their mobility, driving to medical appointments, grappling with insurance and finances – and all the while trying to deal with his or her own grief, fear, and anxiety. From time to time the caregiver wonders, "Who will take care of *me?*" Both patient and caregiver are physically, emotionally, and relationally bereft, while yearning for some meaningful bonding. (Signpost #6 on the Path of Suffering.) The "WE," feeling depleted and needy, begins to yield its head, demanding energy. It's so much easier to elicit negative energy – registering a complaint, expressing resentment, needling the other by being impatient and short-tempered. In these situations the negativity intensifies. Often-times the couple can put on a good front for others, but in private, negative energy dominates.

When Alan was dying from an advanced heart condition and diabetes, he and Judy, his wife of 45 years, experienced this. Each felt unappreciated, resentful, and, at times, angry and fearful. The intensity of emotions frightened them, and their negative responses filled each of them with guilt and shame. Judy recalls one night when Alan complained about everything she tried to do. "The dinner's bland, it has no taste. You know I hate broccoli. Who could eat this?" Alan spit his food in his napkin, dropped his fork with a bang, and shoved the plate aside. Provoked, Judy grabbed the dish and flung it in the sink, shattering it, the remains of Alan's dinner splashing onto the counter, wall, and curtains. That woke them both up. They were shocked and frightened. What was happening to them? Who were they becoming? The bottom line was that the "WE" was starving. It demanded energy, and energy is what it got – negative energy.

In a negative climate there's a serious limitation to the depth and breadth of any conversation. We become defensive, less open to whatever the other has to say. This is why I always urge people to make a strong conscious effort, with the help of God, to fast from any negativity, as described in Chapter 17 (Fasting from Being Preoccupied, Emotionally Withdrawn, Indifferent, Negative, Abusive, Critical, Ungrateful, Demanding, Self-Absorbed, Resistant, Uncooperative, Mistrustful, Insensitive, Punitive, Judgmental, Discouraging, Impatient) and, instead, to deliberately engage in positive relational behaviors. Intentional positive energy given to the other fuels a relationship that becomes more open, and each party becomes less defensive. All of this expands the fertile patch within, opening the "WE" to God's love. And the more love we receive, the more we have to give away. This is why I constantly encourage families who are dealing with these challenges to make it a point to "Do Little Things with Great Love." These activities warm the emotional climate, open the heart, and prepare the soil for the loving conversations that need to be had.

As the positivity increases, the climate of the relationship goes from warm, to warmer, to hot. The destructive inner noise becomes quiet and more intimate levels of conversation become possible. Instead of talking superficially about people, events, and things, all of which divert attention from the more significant issues, a warm environment fosters discussion of deeper thoughts and feelings. As this interpersonal dynamic becomes integrated into the relationship, loved ones can begin to share the ways that being on the Path of Suffering has changed them. They can have candid loving conversations about their greatest fears or regrets, their hopes and dreams - those realized and those lost. They can examine what life has taught them, and profess what they've meant to one another. Forgiveness can be granted and accepted, wounds healed. Memories savored. As a result of their enlightenment along the Path of

Suffering, they can explain how they've changed, who God has become for them, and where they've come to see the hand of God in their lives. Sharing their experience of God deepens the faith life of the other, as well as the relationship between them.

In short, the elephant in the room has to be acknowledged. Not only acknowledged, but embraced. Explored. In doing so you deflate the balloon of anxiety surrounding it, and the frightening power it has over you dramatically decreases. Each person feels more understood, less lonely and afraid.

We've opened the door a crack, and a hint of sun shines in. In the next chapter we'll throw back the door and cast a beam of light into all the dark corners. What are the bigger issues we need to discuss – and how can we address them?

CHAPTER 25

Facing the Elephant

MOST FAMILIES I deal with begin by tip-toeing around the elephant in the sick room. Barbara and I saw this when we visited Kathy (Chapter 20) in Brigham Women's Hospital in Boston. Kathy and her 20 year old daughter Lily were very close. They could talk about anything – except Kathy's impending death. Once I stood in Kathy's story, the reason for this reticence became clear. As a teenager Kathy had lost her own mother to cancer. She could still recall the pain of that time, a time when she was reaching her own womanhood, when the bond between mother and daughter had begun to blossom in new and deeper ways. Kathy desperately wanted to shield Lily from this pain, and agonized over the sad irony of history repeating itself.

Kathy's 26 year-old son, James, when alone with his mother, addressed her death, head-on. Despite an awkward and difficult start, he pressed forward, and mother and son discussed how each felt about her dying. Once the elephant was placed in full view they were able to speak freely about who they'd been for one another, the memories they shared, and gifts they'd treasured. James said it was a liberating and intimate conversation – one he will never forget.

Still, Kathy couldn't bring herself to discuss this with Lily. Instead of serving to protect her, the elephant in the room only added stress. There was a constant undercurrent of tension and restraint that exhausted both women. Later, mother and daughter would say that they'd wanted to discuss what they were both going through – in fact, they knew they had to. But no one wanted to be the one to expose the elephant.

When I visited I could sense their unspoken need. As I took it all in I looked between them and said, "The escalator of life moves pretty fast, doesn't it? "

Kathy nodded. "Faster than I'd like it to." She and Lily exchanged a look and both teared up. Lily took her mother's hand.

"We're all on the escalator, Kath," I said. "From the day we're born. All headed toward a more complete oneness with God and all that is. Death is the gateway to this deeper knowing. And while it feels like a separation, it's actually a communion. When we die we become one with God."

I gazed at Lily, who seemed to be holding her breath. "Lily? " I asked. "Where do you think God is?" Unable to speak, she glanced upward, blinking back tears. "God is here," I said, placing my hand on my chest. I pointed to her. "And here. God dwells inside each of us. So when your mom dies she becomes one with God, in perfect love. So where will she be?"

Lily patted her chest with one hand, squeezed her mom's hand with the other. "Inside me," she whispered.

"She'll be a living and loving presence within you, Lily, loving you in new and deeper ways. Your mom will be able to bring you closer to God's love."

"Yes, I will," Kathy said. "I'll never leave you, Lily, not really. I'll just keep on loving you, more and more."

"And I'll keep on loving you!" Lily answered. The two embraced, crying.

But these weren't tears of sadness.

The elephant had left the room. There was suddenly space to breathe. Kathy and Lily continued to, ever so gently, pursue this conversation. All it took was an entré to get past the initial tentativeness and fear.

Jim, one of my parishioners, shared another example of how painful it can be to avoid discussing an impending death, particularly when a child is involved. When Jim was 9 his 49 year old mother died of breast cancer. While Jim knew she was sick, he and his brother did not understand the seriousness of the illness until she was gone. Jim explained, "For most of my life I've harbored an aching sadness due to my mother's death from cancer nearly 50 years ago. In addition to the indescribable pain of losing Mom, I felt neglected and overlooked because she had not left me a journal, a diary or even a letter with guidance as to how to live without her. Over the years, whenever I saw books like *The Last Lecture*, I would be jealous of the surviving children because they had at least been given some lasting wisdom from their dying parents."

Jim's aunt Frances cared for Jim and his brother through the years, and had the boys stay with her at her cottage each summer. It wasn't until Frances was dying that she told Jim about the time leading up to his mother's death in which his mother asked Frances to care for her boys and nurture them with the love she herself would be unable to provide. Jim learned that his mother had indeed tried her best to leave a legacy of love with her young sons through the care of her sister. Frances had carried this out in a myriad of ways, and Jim and his brother always felt loved and cared for. The unfortunate part of the story is that Jim had to wait almost half a century to learn that his mother had arranged it. How many years of longing and regret might have been avoided if there had been open communication between them?

How I Open the Door to Loving Conversations (Exposing the Elephant)

I'm going to share with you the essence of and my doorway into these conversations. As a spiritual guide, and often a much more objective third party participant, it's important to remember that you won't necessarily be able to replicate this approach in exactly the same way – the dynamic between family members is much more complex. However, I'm also going to share a tool that families have used very successfully to initiate conversations that may initially have felt impossible - just too difficult, too upsetting, or too frightening. This imposed cloak of silence becomes just one more burden for everyone to carry. And it's a frighteningly lonely place for both the patient and family to be.

GENTLE PROBING QUESTIONS

The first thing I do is to strive to understand the patient's world. It's critically important to *really* listen empathetically before sharing what *I* think and feel. It's natural to begin with some small talk about their day-to-day routine, some straight-forward questions about treatment. This readies the soil. Then I'll ask, *"So, what's happening physically? What is your body telling you?"* I listen, not only to the facts, but to their tone of voice, facial expression, gestures, body language. Then I'll read it back to them, often incorporating a bit of what I think I heard that they didn't verbalize. If they're reticent to share, or seemingly not in touch with their physical state of being I might ask, *"What are the doctors and nurses telling you? What non-verbal messages are you picking up on?"* Again, I pay close attention, and read back what I hear. By demonstrating that I listened to their responses acutely, with what I call "all my antennae up," I affirm their reality. They feel relief at having someone understand this strange and perplexing world they find themselves in. This establishes a kind of trust that encourages them to begin to let down their guard even more.

Then, I invite them to get in touch with their emotions and feelings by asking, *"You have a lot of time on your hands – what do you spend most of your time thinking about? What are you feeling?"* This elicits a wide range of responses: "I wish I could just get out of here." "I'm always full of anxiety." "I feel stuck." "I know I'm not getting better." The important thing is not to, in any way, deny what they're saying. The natural impulse is to reassure, to say that it's probably not as bad as all that, that they look good, that there's always some new treatment, etc. etc. But that only serves to discourage further conversation, and to make them feel as though no one really understands their reality.

Here's an example of the way I respond when the dying let me in a little bit.

Fr. Tom: *So, what's happening physically? What's your body saying to you?*

Patient: *There's a heaviness that I feel. I have no energy.*

Fr. Tom: *So, you're really tired...*

Patient: *In more ways than one. Physically tired. But tired of everything.*

Fr. Tom: *Those feelings are normal, natural. Everyone experiences them on the Path of Suffering.*

Patient: *It doesn't feel natural. I feel stuck.*

Fr. Tom: *Let's look at the Path of Suffering so that you have a frame, a context for what you're experiencing.* (I take out a copy of the Path of Suffering, chapter 2.) *Let's "walk" it together so we can better deal with this, so you don't feel so alone in the experience. As we go through each signpost along the path, let me know if you've experienced what I'm describing. You may have spent a lot of time at a particular signpost, or maybe you haven't been there yet.*

At this point we read each signpost along the Path of Suffering. Invariably, at signpost one (dealing with overwhelming thoughts and emotions) whomever I'm working with begins to nod emphatically. "Yes!" they say. "Yes! I've been there! That's exactly what it's like!"

I'm always struck by what appears to be the excitement people express when they see themselves and their experience on the page. "Finally," they exclaim, "Someone understands what I'm going through!"

I always ask for couples or family members to go through the Path of Suffering together, especially since it's easy to focus on the patient and to forget that the primary caregiver is also on the Path of Suffering.

One afternoon I was outside the church when Art cycled by. He and his wife Andrea were former parishioners who I hadn't seen in quite a while. I said hello, asked him how life was treating him. He told me that Andrea had been diagnosed with COPD, and that the disease was nearing its final stages. Clearly they were struggling, not only with the disease, but with all of the issues that come along with it. "I'd love to be able to meet with the two of you," I said. "Talk this through."

"That would be great, Father," Art replied.

Soon afterward I stopped by their house. Andrea was sitting in her chair, hooked up to the oxygen that helped her breathe, Art beside her. I asked Andrea how she was doing and she told me about the disease, the restrictions of it, the pain and effort required to breathe. I told her that I had a "tool" I wanted to share with them – what I sometimes call "a clothes-line" on which their experiences could be hung, looked at, discussed. And I walked them through the Path of Suffering. "If any part of this captures your experience – either what you've already been through, or are going through now, let's talk about it." I made a point of explaining that it wasn't only Andrea on the Path of Suffering, but that Art too was walking right alongside, dealing with similar emotional struggles, negative or anxious thoughts, even spiritual darkness. This piqued Art's attention.

As we walked by each signpost they recognized the landscape well – it was a path well-traveled by both of them. When we came to Signpost #6 – Feeling Tired, Stuck, and Relationally Depleted – Andrea suddenly became animated. Her whole body posture changed. "Yes!" she said. "That's exactly where I am!" It was clear that the description of this sign-post captured her present life - "being sick of the whole thing" – the appointments, the treatments – and the energy it took to try to relate to others. Her feelings were validated and she finally felt understood. Articulating her reality was a form of empathetic listening, giving voice to what she'd been experiencing.

Then I looked at Art. "Art, did you hear what Andrea was saying? "

"Yes," he said, a range of emotions playing across his face.

"And what about you? " I asked him. "What are you experiencing? " Art hesitated. "Go ahead," I said.

He sighed. "Yes," he responded quietly, "I'm going through all the same things. But, who am I to feel that way? I'm not the one who's sick. I feel guilty admitting it. I should be strong for her."

"Art," I said, "You don't need to be strong for her. You need to be *real* with her. That's the doorway to intimacy, the stuff of open, honest, loving communication. When you don't share your thoughts and emotions with Andrea, her perception is that you're *not* on the Path of Suffering with her. You're off on the sidelines and she's going through it alone."

Art looked at his wife. "I *am* tired of the whole thing. And a lot of the time I feel too exhausted to relate. But I *do* love you and I try to be there for you."

Andrea's eyes welled up. "I didn't realize..." She reached out for him. "I love you so much. I love you..." She repeated it over and over again.

Art said, "Honey, thank you. I haven't heard that...those words of love... in months and months..."

The two of them cried, and held each other. A well-spring of intimacy had opened between them. I stood and said a quiet goodbye. As I got to the door, I turned. "Thank you for inviting me into your world. Now remember, please, you don't have to be strong, or hold back in order to protect the other. Keep the communication coming – open, honest, and loving."

Now, granted, given my background and training, it's often easier for me to facilitate these initial conversations than it is for family members. The more emotionally connected each person is to the other, the harder it can be to begin a conversation about painful eventualities that dramatically affect them both. In addition, couples or close family members have long established patterns of communication and well-defined roles that are being challenged. One or both may be resistant to a conversation that needs to be had. Many couples avoid it altogether, preferring to tiptoe around the elephant in the room. In my experience, this is a source of great regret later on.

So, how can one Soul Partner begin? Look at the following exchange. It is essentially the same conversation that I had in all the important ways – but, the warmth of the words, the heartfelt honesty makes this conversation less clinical and more intimate.

Jan: *How are you feeling, Dave?*

Dave: *Phew. Lousy. Don't feel like getting up. No energy.*

Jan: *You're really tired…*

Dave: *Yeah. Tired of everything. I feel shitty. It never gets better.* (looks away)

Jan: (Puts her arms around him.) *Honey, I wish that by putting my arms around you, I could somehow take away your pain. But, I can't. So, the least I can do is try to stand in your world with you…to try to really understand what you're going through – in my own way I'm going through it too. We're in this together. I know it's hard to talk about…but, I read something called the Path of Suffering – and it really resonated with me. I'd like for the both of us to read it. Talk about it.*

Dave: *I don't know…what difference would it make?*

Jan: *Let's just see…it can't hurt…it might help us talk about what's happening to the both of us…*

Facilitating Loving Conversations - Stephie's Story

Sometimes one family member can facilitate this process for others. Stephie came to me because her father, Nino, was dying of cancer. Besides dealing with the grief and sense of loss that Nino's impending death was causing, Stephie was shocked and saddened by the apparent change in his personality. He had become angry and nasty, taking out his frustration on Stephie's mom. At the same time friends and family were "cheering him on" telling him he had to keep fighting, that he could beat this disease. They'd force him to eat, to "build his strength." Their well-meaning efforts contradicted what he was experiencing. Nino felt an ever-increasing sense of isolation and resentment.

At Stephie's urging I called Nino, who lived out of state. I asked him what his body was telling him – he replied that he knew he was dying despite the fact that no one had told him so. I talked with him about the Path of Suffering, validating his experience and standing in his world with him. Then I told him, "Nino, you have little time and a lot of work to do." I explained that his calling and responsibility, his real life's mission was the work of loving. His voice suddenly became more animated. Finally, someone had been real with him. Finally, there was something of value he could accomplish. I explained that I wanted him to fast from negativity and to begin to do little things with great love. But he still was reticent about bringing up the topic of his death. He wanted, first and foremost, to protect his family from it.

So, I also spoke to Stephie about becoming her father's guide. She tried to enlist the help of her siblings, encouraging them all to have an honest conversation with Dad about his condition and their feelings about it. Her brother was furious – how dare she rob their father of hope? He wasn't going to have any such conversation. But Stephie formed an alliance with her sister, both agreeing that what would help their dad most was support in his mission to love. Stephie sat with him, and told him, "Dad, I'm so sorry you're really sick. It stinks – you're hurting and I'm so sorry I can't fix it." This opened the door to some honest dialogue. After establishing this mutual trust Stephie took it a step further, helping him to say the things she knew he wanted to say, but didn't know how. "I know how difficult it is to sometimes say the things that need to be said. But there's no need to try to "protect" one another. Maybe you need to talk to Mom. Tell her how you really feel. You just don't know how much time you have left."

Nino left the hospital for hospice care at home where he and his wife celebrated a bittersweet 50th anniversary. It was an effort, but Nino smiled and spoke words of thanks and appreciation to all of their guests. When the party ended Nino lay in bed with his eyes closed. As his wife was caring for him he opened his eyes and quietly sang, *"You'll never know how much I really love you...You'll never know how much I really care..."* Stephie's mom cried and she and Nino embraced. It was an uncharacteristically demonstrative expression of his feelings, a real stretch beyond his comfort zone. The affect on his wife and family was profound and lasting.

Establishing a Communication Commitment

The types of interactions I've just described are by no means "one-and-done" encounters. What I've outlined is simply a way to break the ice, to begin a dialogue that will deepen and grow when both parties commit to the process. In order to build on this, to intensify the intimacy and level of sharing, I ask couples and other loved ones to form what I call a "Communication Commitment." In doing so, *both* parties agree to take responsibility to initiate open, honest, and loving conversations, to embrace the courage it takes to broach difficult subjects, to practice empathetic listening, and to address the issues they're facing in solidarity and love. They pledge to acknowledge the suffering of the other along the path, to fast from negativity, and to consistently "do little things with great love."

CHAPTER 26

Beginning to Discuss Life and Death Issues - The Art of Being Real

INTIMACY IS THE art of being real with those we care about - with sensitivity and love. At a time when so much has been lost, engaging in an intimate conversation – even a very difficult conversation – can form a bond and alliance that makes both parties feel fully alive. Intimate sharing builds bridges between the isolated places that we tend to suffer in alone. These conversations forge a meeting of minds and hearts that dispels loneliness and desperation. What a privilege to enter this sacred common ground, to gently take on, respect, and honor the thoughts, feelings, and wishes of another.

This process of emotional give-and-take demands tremendous vulnerability, unfailing trust, and deep faith, especially when the conversation centers around the emotional minefields surrounding sickness, dying, and death. This is why we suggested, in the last chapter, that you form an intentional Communication Commitment in order to sustain you through the process. Before addressing the highly charged topics in this chapter, it's helpful to recommit to your Communication Commitment. Knowing that you're in it together can make all the difference. Make a conscious intention, in faith, to open yourself up to this wellspring of the Spirit inside you. You've been emptied by suffering, but our loving, merciful God will fill you, so that God's unconditional love, forgiveness, and healing can spill into and inform every exchange.

ATTRIBUTES OF GOOD COMMUNICATION
Communication is an art that must be learned and practiced. Too often we confuse talking with communicating. We talk *at* rather than *with* one

another. When topics to be discussed are steeped in powerful emotions, tied to past hurts, present issues, and future losses, the process becomes even more challenging. Therefore it's crucial to enter the process mindfully and to learn some of the basics on how to engage in a meaningful loving exchange.

We've already discussed the importance of creating a warm climate, fasting from negative behaviors, and doing little things with great love. These contribute to the best environment for loving conversations. Now let's look at some of the basic skills that allow for the art of communication.

Some people are naturally better at being able to articulate their thoughts and feelings clearly, to put abstract feelings into words, to keep talking their way into knowing. These are often also people with a willingness to disclose parts of their inner world to others.

Regardless of how public or private a person we are, we can all learn to communicate on deeper levels. An impending death exposes our vulnerability, and suddenly there is little to lose by holding on to inhibitions. In light of that, there are some techniques we can all practice to empower more meaningful conversation that can build bridges, break down walls, and enrich our relationships.

ACTIVE LISTENING: SPEAK – LISTEN - SPEAK

As a counselor, this is a technique I've taught married couples for years. In order to understand our partner, we have to *really* listen. We can't listen when we're constantly mining our own brains for our next response, interjecting every time something is said that sets us off balance. We have to step back from any notion of "being right" or of "winning someone over."

After the two of you name the issue you want to discuss, decide who'll be the speaker and who'll be the listener.

The **speaker** begins, verbalizing her/his thoughts and feelings on the issue. "I" statements are stressed (rather than "you" statements.) It might be helpful to begin the conversation with some of the following:

- *Right now, here's what concerns me:*
- *I'm feeling_____.*
- *I get confused when_____.*
- *I wish that_____*   • *I regret_____*

- *I'm torn between_____.*
- *What I'd like to see happen is____.*
- *I'm sad, angry, frightened because__.*
- *I'm sorry for_____.*

The speaker takes as long as need be, speaking until she/he is satisfied that the issue has been thoroughly explained from her/his perspective.

When you're the **listener** you may not interrupt or interject, but you may ask for clarification: *In what sense? Tell me more about that. How does that make you feel? Can you give me an example?* Your only job is to listen to what your partner is saying, and to strive to understand the world from their legitimate viewpoint. Hear the other out, completely. When the speaker is finished, reiterate what you've heard to ensure that you've grasped your partner's meaning, without any editorial comments. *"What I hear you saying is that..." "Am I missing anything?" "Did I hear you? "*Your job is not to contradict, dispute, or challenge the other's point of view. The goal is to stay in your partner's world until she/he is satisfied that you understand. If you missed anything or misunderstood, the speaker will then clarify, and the process is repeated before changing roles.

This takes patience and practice. But when approached with fidelity to the process, the results can be life-changing. Unresolved issues can be ironed out as each of you understands the other's perspective. There is nothing more powerful than knowing you've been heard - *really* heard - by someone you care about. Once you've heard and understood each other's point of view, the result is solidarity and mutual compassion. You can apply this process to any and all of the topics that follow.

Topics to be Addressed

One way to dispel some of the tension around the difficult issues is to lay them out on the table. This book will help you do that. Whether you're the patient, loved one, or caregiver, you can begin as simply and honestly as this: *"I feel there are a lot of things we need to discuss – but I don't really know where to start. It feels a little scary to me. Maybe we could look at this chapter together? Begin to talk about one topic at a time? Let the book lead the way?"*

The best way to deflate fears is to address and discuss them. It's important to be able to put fears in perspective so that both partners will be free enough to move beyond them in order to talk about the many other life-giving and life-changing topics that need to be explored and shared.

Read through the following list of common fears together, then agree to only approach one of these fears at a time. Your feelings may change as the escalator moves forward, so give yourselves permission to revisit these topics as the physical, emotional, and spiritual landscape changes. Make a pact to agree to active listening, following the guidelines outlined earlier.

Fear of:

- **The unknown** • **Abandonment** • **Pain and great suffering**
- **Becoming a burden physically and/or** • **Losing One's Dignity**
  financially

Now is the time when the tire hits the road – where you begin to apply everything we've explored thus far. Keep in mind that, where you find yourself on the Path of Suffering will color your response to each issue. It's helpful to go back and read through the Path of Suffering (Chapter 2) again, with an eye for the dominant emotion elicited at each signpost. That emotion will affect the way you respond to each fear on this discussion list.

If you discover that the prospect of addressing any of these causes you to withdraw, to shut down, become angry or depressed, or catapults you into either the past or the future, consider contemplating the "Prison of Self" (Chapter 8) again. If you experience a compulsion to control, the best way through it to freedom *is to extend yourself in love to others.* Begin to reflect on the ways God has supported you through your "EKG" of life, through all the ups and downs. Take stock of your faith, reflect on the balance between your false and true selves (the Fulcrum, Chapter 3). Create an inventory of all you've been grateful for. Embrace the spiritual practices that help you to know God in the deepest recesses of your heart. Reach outside yourself by focusing on others - doing little things with great love. Be gentle and tolerant with yourself and others. Accept the intense feelings and then let them go. Quietly surrender expectations of what you think others ought to do for you, and accept whatever they can provide with a grateful heart. If you've practiced meditation you'll discover that the same process can be used to own, and at the same time, surrender any negative or stressful ponderings. As you practice this, you'll gradually adapt to each "new normal" where reality, hope, and acceptance meet and transformation takes place. All of this nurtures the bittersweet freedom necessary to prepare for death in a loving, intentional way.

DISCUSSING AND ASSUAGING YOUR FEARS

There are a number of fears often expressed by the dying. What all of these fears have in common is this – they are *all* rooted in the diminishment of the ego/body self (how I define myself in terms of my roles, abilities, accomplishments, relationships). Look back at the Fulcrum in Chapter 3. If we're deeply rooted in the spirit self, feeling one with all that is, and one with God, we feel secure in the fact that we are deeply loved, and this tempers our fears. We're all born with the knowledge of the spirit self within us – at some level we all understand this sacred solidarity. But without intentionally nurturing the spirit self, the ego dominates. *The defense of the ego is what produces anxiety and fear.*

Let's be clear – the concerns addressed below are legitimate and need to be honored and explored – never negated. However, when we're living exclusively through the ego we drastically inflate our anxieties until they dominate our lives. Easing into conversations about these topics helps to "let the air out of the balloon" of these fears.

FEAR OF THE UNKNOWN

The road ahead is a mystery – from the twists and turns of the disease and its effects on day-to-day living, to questions of exactly how and when death will occur. And, of course, what reality on the other side of the grave will be like. There are no answers to these questions and so our sense of security is threatened and illusion of control destroyed. If we haven't done the work of nurturing the spirit self, the ego will assert itself, drive us toward seeking answers and desperately try to control the situation.

So, what is the best way to share and discuss a fear of the unknown? Conversations that connect us to "all that is" are soothing and helpful. While the ego self insists on its own autonomy, its own individualistic identity, the spirit self reminds us that we're one with all life in a seamless, timeless way. We're connected to those who've gone before us, and share in their experiences. (In the Catholic Christian tradition we refer to this as the "Communion of Saints.") We're united with all people through our common humanity and the Spirit of God that flows through all of us. The same life force that brings flowers to bud, bloom, and fade runs through our veins. Being a pilgrim on this sacred journey of life can conjure deep joy in the profound bittersweet experience of living this mystery.

When Arlene was dying of liver cancer, the endless questions about when, why, and how tormented her, filling her with anxiety. She found herself in a state of constant nervous irritability, unable to focus on the present moment or respond mindfully to those around her. After snapping at her husband Bill for the hundredth time she burst into tears. "Arlene," Bill said, "Please, talk to me. What's going on inside you? "

"I'm scared," Arlene cried, "Of everything! What's going to happen to me, today? Tomorrow? What will happen when I'm gone? "

Bill took her by the hand and pulled her close. "Come here, Ar," he said. They sat by the window that overlooked her beloved garden. "Here's what I know for sure. However this disease unfolds, I'll be here with you. God will be with you too." He patted his heart. "You'll always be right here." He kissed her hair and she tucked her head beneath his chin. "None of us knows when we'll die. But whether you're here or in the hospital, if I'm literally there beside you or not, we're still together." Arlene nuzzled closer. Bill lifted her chin so they looked into one another's eyes. "And not only that, Arlene," he said softly. "When you go, you take my heart with you. We're one, now and forever." The two of them cried, sighed, and stared out at the garden. Bill thought of all the times he'd watched her planting and weeding, trimming, and cutting fresh flowers. "Your spirit fills this place Arlene. When your body goes, the heart and soul of you stays. I'll cherish that."

This conversation radically changed their relationship. Arlene later told Bill that she'd never loved him more than during that brief but powerful exchange. Months after Arlene died, when Bill shared all of this with me, he explained how that garden continued to be a source of strength for him. "I'm telling you, Fr. Tom," he said. "I feel her presence there – it's as if she lives on in the flowers, in the earth itself." He shook his head, incredulous. "What a gift..."

We all need to be reminded of the eternal nature of our relationships, with those we love and with the world around us. An affirmation of that helps reinforce our inherent solidarity with all that is, which reduces the fear and isolation of the unknown.

FEAR OF ABANDONMENT

As the lives of those around you go on, you may feel as though you've been left behind. You spend more time alone, and your world seems to shrink. The days drag on and your isolation begins to give way to loneliness. This causes you to become more needy, clinging to a spouse or other loved one, demanding more time and energy than he/she can realistically give. Anxieties increase. You may even fear dying alone.

Expressing the fear of abandonment helps dispel it. The patient might say, "Honey, I know you need to go to work. But I'm struggling spending so much time alone. My mind races and I start to worry. I'm not trying to make you feel bad. But I need some help in working this through."

This honest admission opens the door to empathy - and some practical solutions.

Loved ones can set up a regular schedule of visits and phone calls from family, friends, and caregivers, bringing some structure and predictability to the patient's days. Facetime or Skype is another way to connect with others on an agreed-upon schedule.

However, being proactive in reaching out is even more beneficial. Writing a note to a friend or family member, sending a greeting card or thank you note maintains a loving connection and fills empty hours with positive gestures of love and appreciation. Initiating email or phone calls inquiring about loved ones shifts the focus away from self. Consider pouring over old photographs of loved ones, including a memory you've penned on the back. Slip them in an envelope and send them off. If this is physically challenging, enlist the help of a friend, a volunteer from your church community, or home health aide. It's empowering to take the initiative, even if assistance is required. This is another form of doing little things with great love, intentionally opening yourself to God, and transforming loneliness to solitude.

Engaging in spiritual practices also shifts the focus away from the ego and allows the perceived emptiness to be filled with the awareness of God's presence. Consider reading and reflecting on the following scripture passages. Each speaks to God's presence in the face of loneliness.

Isaiah 41:10
"Fear not, I am with you;
Be not dismayed; I am your God."

Matthew 28:20
"I am with you always, until the end of the age."

Psalm 28:7
"The LORD is my strength and my shield, in whom my heart trusted and found help."

John 14:27
"Peace I leave with you, my peace I give to you. Not as the world gives do I give it to you. Do not let your hearts be troubled or afraid."

FEAR OF PAIN AND GREAT SUFFERING

When fears and anxieties grab hold we tend to waver between control and surrender. Our natural response to pain, or even the threat of pain, is a defensive one. We need to control the physical discomfort – and that's legitimate. But, at the same time we need to surrender the fear and anxiety that often accompanies physical pain so as not to exacerbate that pain with emotional and mental suffering. In addition, remaining firmly rooted in the spirit self helps remind us that we're so much more than a physical being. Being involved in gentle spiritual practices can temper not only the fear of pain, but our response to it.

Despite the fact that doctors have a wide range of techniques and medications to treat physical pain, this continues to be a source of great fear amongst the dying. It seems, however, that fear of physical pain in the terminally ill is often inflated. Emotional or spiritual suffering can be interpreted as physical pain, in which case pain medication seems ineffective.

Another aspect of this quandary is that many doctors are uncomfortable confronting the issue of dying with their patients, and in circumventing that conversation, find it easier to persist in hopeless, often painful and invasive procedures and treatments.

It's clear that having a frank conversation with your medical team about the reality of your condition and the ramifications in terms of pain is essential. This is another instance of how a Communication Commitment can be powerful. Arrange for a meeting between Communication Commitment partners and the doctor in charge. Together you can establish an understanding in regard to pain and treatment options. Some important straightforward questions to ask:

- Will this treatment cure my disease or prolong my quality of life? If so, how?
- If you or a family member were in my shoes, what treatment would you opt for, given the circumstances? (Doctors often decline aggressive end-of-life treatment for themselves.)
- If we suspend this treatment, what can I expect to happen, and on what timeline?
- What medications or other treatments are available for pain and how effective are they?
- Can I monitor my own need for pain medication, and if so, what are the consequences of that?

I highly recommend that you and your loved one or caregiver do some homework prior to a medical consult. Knowing the options can broaden the conversation. An excellent resource is *Dying Well* by Dr. Ira Byock, which answers many questions regarding pain management that can inform your conversation. Knowing that your care-giver, loved ones, and medical team understand your legitimate concerns in terms of pain management provides a level of security that helps allay this fear.

Also, establishing a warm relationship with nursing staff who are responsible for the front line of your care and talking with them about your fears can be helpful. These are women and men who responded to a calling to alleviate the suffering of others, so much so that they made it their career. A willingness to be vulnerable with them (rather than trying to be stoic) will ensure that your pain is carefully monitored and treated accordingly. It is always more effective to "get ahead of the pain" by using medication preemptively than it is to "chase" pain with medication once the pain has a hold on you. I always say, "It's better to get on the horse than to chase the horse." Being forthright with nursing staff can help in this regard.

Additionally, there's evidence that many patients respond to alternative pain treatments, such as acupuncture or massage, which not only can reduce physical discomfort, but also the anxiety and fear that contribute to suffering. Without a doubt, caring for the whole person, and in particular, for the spirit self, is a powerful antidote. A loved one can secure alternative therapy and supportive pastoral care in order to help alleviate a patient's pain. Taking the patient's hand, providing a gentle shoulder rub or head massage, helps root them firmly in the present – it's hard to fear future pain while experiencing the nurturance of a family member of friend. A loving massage is a good time for a loving conversation:

Caregiver: *How does this feel?*
Patient: *Ahh...it feels good. But, my legs still ache. I don't know what I'll do as this gets worse. I don't think I can stand it...*
Caregiver*: Try to relax and just soak up my touch. Let's not give this moment away running into the future. No one knows what tomorrow holds. I just love being able to offer you a tender touch. You can always count on me for that. You're never going to be alone in this.*
Patient: *But what if...*
Caregiver: *Let's talk to your doctor about it. If we need to we can adjust your medication. I was thinking about acupuncture - finding a therapist to work with you on your pain. Relax you. And, Fr. Tom can come and give you the sacrament of the sick...*
Patient: *As long as I know you're here.*
Caregiver: *And when I'm not, I'll be near enough to jump in and troubleshoot for you. You know that...*

In the Catholic faith it's customary to receive the sacrament of the sick (not to be confused with "last rites.") This spiritual response to pain can be a balm to the afflicted by imparting the grace and strength of the Holy Spirit. When I anoint patients with the sacrament of the sick, I always share with them the prayer of St. Francis de Sales:

"Do not look forward to what may happen tomorrow; the same everlasting Father who cares for you today will take care of you tomorrow and every day. Either He will shield you from suffering, or He will give you unfailing strength to bear it. Be at peace, then, put aside all anxious thoughts and imaginations."

I ask them to keep the prayer nearby, to pray it every time fear and anxiety threaten to overwhelm them. Recite it as an act of faith, even when their fears seem insurmountable and their world appears to be closing in. The very act of repeating the words as a life-giving mantra can go a long way toward releasing the fears that can grow and spread like wild fire.

FEAR OF BECOMING A BURDEN, PHYSICALLY AND/OR FINANCIALLY
We all realize that our resources are limited. That the time, energy, and finances of a family can go only so far. Worries about stretching or expending these resources are legitimate. For the patient, the idea of causing the family to become overburdened or financially strapped only adds emotional suffering to the pain of the disease. For the family, anxiety and exhaustion sometimes translate into resentment and guilt. Therefore, the fear of becoming a burden needs to be addressed in a straightforward, pragmatic way - both to relieve the patient's worries and to strategize on the most life-giving and realistic ways of utilizing the resources at hand.

Often, the patient will insist on doing things independently that are no longer feasible. Their desire to not become burdensome can actually cause great stress for the very people the patient is trying to spare. So as not to "bother" anyone, the patient might be resistant to help - not asking for assistance in getting out of bed, toileting, or getting dressed. Not only does this stance cause needless worry for caregivers, but it is, moreover, a stance of control. It can lead to accidents and injuries, making patient care even more complicated. I always urge patients to ask a question that can address, to some extent, their fear of becoming a burden. This question can be a real gift to the caregiver or loved one, and it is this: *How can I help you help me?* And then, I ask the patient to be open and cooperative in regard to the caregiver's response. In fact, this is an opportunity to become what Jesus referred to as "the least among us," to allow loved ones and caregivers to be the hands of a healing, loving God.

But more often than not, patients hold onto control, and this prevents them from appreciating the efforts of others. *"Let yourself be loved!"* is another thing I tell people. It's amazing how hard it is for us to submit to the working of God through others. As patients, we make it so much easier for our caregivers when we willingly surrender to their care.

The fear of becoming a financial burden is a legitimate one in our culture. With the constantly rising cost of healthcare, treatments, hospitalization, and medication, a family without significant resources can find themselves financially strapped. Of course, long term planning before an illness strikes can go a long way to assuaging these fears. Having a health insurance plan, long-term care insurance, a network and support system beyond the immediate family can prevent burnout. But, in the absence of these, many families benefit by consulting with an objective third party who can help in addressing these concerns. A trusted lawyer can advise on the best ways to protect financial assets, and a social worker, case manager or other medical professional can guide families through the sometimes complex network of insurance benefits and caregiving options. Sometimes, however, for a variety of legitimate reasons, many families have not adequately budgeted for the financial demands of a long-term illness. Mounting medical bills, debt, and the prospect of new and ever more costly treatments can add tremendous pressure to an already stressful situation. It can be heart-wrenching for the patient to feel as though the family must choose between top-notch medical treatment and financial viability. One long-time parishioner, when facing this dire reality, chose to take his own life rather than leave his wife of over 50 years with a mountain of debt. His intention was to free them from financial ruin, but his decision left the family permanently traumatized. After all this couple had been through together, he chose an ending that his wife never would have wanted. There was no peace in this final chapter, and the family was tormented with images, worries, and doubts that were never to be fully resolved or healed.

So, what is the answer? I always counsel families to discuss the viability of any extraordinary or excessive treatments that will not result in a cure. Spending great sums of money to extend a life already diminished by serious illness, with no hope of recovery is a futile exercise. My mother, when diagnosed with colon cancer that had spread to the liver, was "given" 12 months to live. Because hers was an incurable condition my mother and the family decided to decline treatment, aside from anything that would help keep her comfortable. She experienced very little pain, and despite the expected 12 month window, lived for 22 months. This was a peaceful time in which my mother enjoyed her family and her home. Ultimately, spending a fortune on costly aggressive treatments or experimental drugs that might prolong her life an extra few months just didn't seem the right choice. An important conversation around these kinds of considerations is critical.

This is *not* to suggest that the criteria around a decision about extending or increasing treatment should be a financial one. But I am suggesting that making thoughtful decisions about the viability of extending life needs to be determined by the quality of life sustained by such treatment. Many times, quality of life can be improved by suspending costly and futile treatments. The list of questions on p.289 (under fear of great pain and suffering) can be used to help make these kinds of decisions, which are entirely personal. Planning advance directives (Chapter 28) can help ensure that the right decisions are made in each individual circumstance.

FEAR OF THE LOSS OF DIGNITY

One of the greatest fears that the terminally ill struggle with is the loss of dignity. On the most basic level, losing control of body functions can make us feel ashamed. What if I can't get to the bathroom by myself? If I have to wear a diaper? We fear being infantilized, feel embarrassed by making public a very private part of personal caretaking. Exposing a loved one or trusted caregiver to the sights and smells associated with this can be demoralizing. No one wants to lose the ability to wash, dress, and feed oneself. Jesus acknowledges this in John 21:18:

> Amen, amen, I say to you, when you were younger, you used to dress your-self and go where you wanted, but when you grow old, you will stretch out your hands, and someone else will dress you and lead you where you do not want to go.

The diminishment that serious illness brings strips us of the very things from which we derive our sense of usefulness and worth. The man who was fastidious in dress, the woman who was highly particular about her hair and make-up can feel undignified when this daily regimen becomes impossible to maintain. Looking in the mirror can be startling – "That's not ME!" Unless we're aware of the role ego plays, our self-consciousness can spiral into negative self-absorption.

What we forget is that every one of us possesses an inherent and immutable dignity in the spirit self – the dignity of who we are in God alone. As we begin to lose the superficial "dignity of the world," becoming "less of who we are," ever more weak and infirm, we find ourselves among those Jesus spoke of in the Beatitudes – the poor in spirit, the "least among us." And it is these "lowly ones" that are closest to the heart of God. It is no accident that Jesus, on his way to Calvary, was stripped and mocked, his suffering displayed in a public forum. Jesus understood that, as a child of God, his dignity and integrity could not, under any circumstances, be destroyed. And we share in that dignity.

While it's important to come to terms with some loss of dignity, and to accept the eventuality of what's likely to occur, it's also helpful to strategize with loved ones to put your mind at ease. If possible, you might relegate assistance with bathing and toileting to a professional caregiver – a home health aide or nurse. The fact that they're trained and accustomed to helping in this way reduces the discomfort and embarrassment. The patient might say to a family member, *"I appreciate your willingness to help me with this. But, if possible, it's just so much more comfortable for both of us to have the home health aide do this. And when they can't, can we find some ways for me to feel less exposed? To maintain some sense of modesty?"* Providing a sheet to partially conceal the patient during changing, and a robe or shawl to cover a johnny coat are small, considerate measures easily taken. Asking the caregiver to avert his/her eyes or to provide a moment of privacy is a reasonable request that should be respected. Also, if incontinence is an issue, an enuresis pad can be used. Rather than having to frequently check to see if an accident has occurred, an alarm alerts the caregiver and bedclothes can be changed immediately. This also helps the caregiver recognize any patterns in order to provide bathroom assistance in anticipation of times when incontinence tends to happen. Humor is another way to "let the air out of the balloon." When Ursula cried in embarrassment when she had an accident that her son Eric had to clean up, Eric said, "Mom, I know you're just getting back at me for those years I resisted potty training." And then, so as not to dismiss her feelings, he leaned over, kissed her forehead and said, "When you love someone, caring for them is a privilege."

Discussing the fears in this chapter can certainly help dispel or at least diminish them. Doing so frees both the patient and caregiver to begin to take a more clear-headed look at the practical decisions that have to be made. In the next chapter we'll look at "getting your house in order" – still another way to bring the satisfaction of closure to the end of life.

CHAPTER 27

Putting Your House in Order

"Put your house in order, because you are going to die; you will not recover."

– 2 Kings 20:1

AT A TIME when emotions are running high, when the family system is under great stress, and the unpredictability of a disease makes it impossible to anticipate what tomorrow holds, it becomes crucial to do the work of putting your house in order. Without a doubt, the highest priority in this regard is to engage in conversations about what matters most – faith, feelings, relationships, gratitude, life-lessons, and saying our goodbyes. But, it can be very difficult to have these intimate conversations when the practical realities of an impending death are pressing in from all sides. So, the sooner these details are addressed, the sooner we can move toward the conversations that really count.

I'd like to tell you about my friend, Fr. Lou, who served as my associate pastor for five years. He went on to lead another parish until his retirement several years ago. It was obvious that he tremendously enjoyed this much-deserved down time, taking advantage of travel opportunities and visits with family and friends until his heart condition dramatically worsened. Still, whenever he was back in Connecticut, Fr. Lou would stay at the rectory with me. We'd watch basketball together, share a meal, a glass of wine, some comfortable conversation. But about a week into his visit, his complexion would begin to turn pasty white and he'd grow weaker by the day until his next blood transfusion. Surgery was out of

297

the question, as odds of him dying during the procedure were higher than gambling on staying alive without it.

We frequently talked about his situation. He knew he was seriously ill, and that the transfusions he was receiving could only buy him so much time. Lou had frank discussions with me, and his sisters and friends about how he wished his treatment, his death, funeral, and burial to unfold. Obviously, he had given all of this a lot of thought, and took into consideration not only his own wishes, but how the plans he made would affect those he loved. Lou embraced the task of "getting his house in order," leaving no stone unturned. He compiled files containing copies of his advance directives, made lists of his insurance policy and bank account numbers, credit card accounts, undertaker, funeral and burial information, all with related contact names and phone numbers. To ensure that we were all on the same page, his sisters and I all received copies. Fr. Lou even gave Barbara the sheet music of a favorite Polish hymn he wanted his sisters to sing at his funeral. He presented all of this with a sense of accomplishment, pleased to be able to take any pressure off of those who had walked through life with him.

Barbara and I were both so impressed with the work he did that we've vowed to begin to put our respective houses in order, gathering the information needed, and updating it each year. What a gift to those who will be caring for us at the end of the day! In fact, whether you're the patient or the caregiver, family member or friend, this is a good time to embrace this work together – in that way making the task seem so much less dire for the patient.

COMPILING ALL NECESSARY PAPERWORK

Perhaps you've already discussed some of these matters. Maybe you've begun the work. Either way, it's extremely important to have all the crucial information, *in writing,* and in a safe place so that your executor, heirs, and family can easily access it. What follows is a list of "must-haves." The list may seem daunting, but it's so much easier to accomplish without the pressure of any critical or time-sensitive decisions that may need to be made.

1. **Appoint someone you trust as your Durable Power of Attorney (POA).** Should you be unable to do so, your POA can do your banking, bill paying, and any financial undertakings on your behalf as specifically designated in the document.

2. **Name a trusted family member or friend as your Medical Power of Attorney.** This appointee becomes your proxy to make medical decisions if and when you're unable to do so. Having a **Living Will** or **Advance Care Directive** lays out your intentions, and helps avoid conflicts between family members who may disagree over medical decisions.

3. **Have a will drawn up or review your existing will.**

4. **If you own a business, have a succession plan.**

5. **Appoint a guardian for any minor children.**

6. **Name an executor to your estate.** This is the person who is responsible for ensuring that your assets and possessions are distributed according to your wishes. They must ensure that all debts are paid and that the remaining assets are distributed as designated in your will. This is a tremendous responsibility, therefore making all necessary account numbers, passwords, documents, etc. readily available is a must. (See list, p.300.)

7. **File or update beneficiary forms** for all bank, life insurance, retirement accounts.

8. **Preplan the funeral.** Establish a budget, and if possible, set funds aside for this purpose. Will there be a wake? How would you like to be clothed and is your outfit set aside? Will there be a funeral service? A burial or a cremation? A gathering afterward?

9. **Life insurance?** If end of life expenses are a concern, purchasing a term life insurance policy might be explored.

10. **Will organs be donated?** To help inform your decision, go to www.organdonor.gov/

11. Provide a list of the following essential information:

- Copies of POA assignment, Advance Directives, Living Will
- Social Security Number
- Most recent tax return
- Deeds to all real estate
- Copies of will, trusts, insurance policies, stock certificates, bonds, annuities
- 401K, IRA's, Retirement account #s
- Bank Account and Mutual Fund Account numbers
- Online banking account numbers and passwords
- Life Insurance Account Numbers
- List of all online recurring payments, payees, pay to account #s, date debited
- Safe deposit box locations, keys, combinations, passwords
- Debt information and account numbers – mortgage, car, utilities, credit cards
- Information for preplanned funeral/burial
- Location of keys to property, cars, storage units, file cabinets, etc.
- Instructions for personal bequests
- Prescription medications on automatic refill, pharmacy information
- Any rented medical equipment, where/how to return it
- List of people to notify upon your death – phone #, email, address for each

If you have a specific attorney, agent, customer representative, or other contact in connection with any of the above, be sure to include these as well.

THE SIMPLIFICATION OF LIFESTYLE

Often, as life is winding down, a great deal of attention and energy is spent by loved ones trying to keep things as close to "normal" as possible.

While the intention is good, the fact is that for the patient, this can produce feelings of sadness, regret, and isolation.

When Myra was in the end stages of life, her husband and daughters went to great lengths to "keep things normal" for her. This included getting her dressed in her usual outfits, fussing with her hair, arranging for her favorite TV shows and meals. Myra felt she needed to keep up a good front for them, and this prevented her from doing some of the important work of dying. What Myra realized was that much of the "stuff" of her previous life had lost its significance. In failing to recognize and embrace Myra's "new normal" her family kept her in a past that no longer existed. Myra had changed. Her priorities and values had been honed and clarified. As the layers of her ego self began to be shed, she felt an inner pull toward things of the spirit. She felt a need to simplify her life, to focus on the significance of this "new normal." Doing so would allow her to gently adjust, to relax into this important transition, and to let go of "what was" with grace and gratitude.

Despite her family's objections, Myra began the process of what I call "the simplification of lifestyle," uncluttering her life so that she would be free from the encumbrances that made it harder for her to let go. Always a bit of a fashionista, Myra had quite a collection of jewelry, both costume and the real deal. She asked for her jewelry to be spread out on the table beside her bed, and slowly and methodically she began to give it away. Daughters and daughters-in law, granddaughters and nieces all received special pieces. Her in-home caregivers went home with pins and necklaces, as did neighbors who brought a covered dish or a bunch of flowers. She had her daughters go through her clothes and shoes, modeling them for her, pressing them to take whatever made them smile. The rest Myra made them promise to box up and send to her church's second-hand store. Her beloved piano, she bequeathed to her grandson, her journals and photo albums to her husband.

After hospice care came in, Myra's meals became simpler, determined primarily by her appetite and energy. The television was mostly turned off in favor of simply *being* with loved ones or listening to music. Less doing, more being.

Metaphorically, all of this represented Myra's gradual transformation from her ego self to her spirit self. In following her instincts she was able to lighten her load for the remainder of her journey. Each "giving away" was a small practice in letting go that would inform and empower her *final* letting go.

Whether we're on the Path of Suffering, facing a terminal illness, or just moving along beyond middle age, getting your house in order along with a gradual and intentional simplification of lifestyle is a valuable exercise. Doing so makes our inevitable final letting go easier. It frees us to focus on what life is really about – being in deep, open, honest conversation with those we love. In the next chapter we'll continue to look at some of the more challenging end-of-life decisions that need to be made in order to help make the transition to the next stage of living that we call death.

CHAPTER 28

Taking Responsibility for Your Care

AFTER SEEING THE moving and thought-provoking Broadway Show starring Sting, titled <u>The Last Ship</u>, both Barbara and I kept revisiting and reflecting on one of the show's tunes, in which the sage and earthy character, Fr. O'Brian, knowing he's close to death, puts forth a song, addressing, head-on, without sentimentality, and with an edge of sarcasm, the question of medical treatment in the face of dying. The good Irish Father comes to the same conclusion as so many others have – that extraordinary measures and extreme treatments to extend life are often worse than the disease itself.

This scenario plays out in real life every day. Lisa and I had been working together when her cancer came back for the second time. Now in the hospital, she found herself in a place where three signposts on the Path of Suffering converged (Interacting with Family and Friends, Navigating Outside Support Systems, and Realizing There's No Turning Back). Crying, she confided that she didn't want any more treatment - she longed for death, to get on with the "next phase." Her husband and sons pressured her to undergo one more round of treatment to extend her life a little longer. With one son's wedding approaching and a grandchild on the way, they reasoned that she had so much to live for. Lisa felt guilty – they'd made it clear they felt she was "giving up," and were disappointed that she'd "lost her fighting spirit." The pressure Lisa felt from both her family and her doctor, combined with the slim hope that this next extreme treatment might buy her a little more time, felt less like hope and more like an extended sentence.

My conversation with Lisa eerily echoed the sentiments of Chester (Chapter 1), when he'd told me, "See, here's how it is – when *you're* sick, you know you're going to feel lousy for a few days or even a week. Then you're gonna get better. But me? Every day I feel sick, and the next day I'm even sicker. And I know there won't be a single morning when I get up stronger than I was the day before. It will just get worse and worse 'til the day I finally die."

What I've seen over the years in dealing with the dying is that when you (or a family member) tries to extend the calendar of your life through desperate means, the result can be a unique kind of hell, incongruent with the life you seek to sustain. The last-ditch treatment, the experimental protocol might yield more days – but the nature and quality of those days can equate to a kind of living death, the hospital room the tomb. Patients may be physically present, but emotionally absent. The situation is often dominated by physical pain and emotional suffering. By holding on we intensify this suffering. (Remember the pencil exercise in Chapter 16? The harder you grasp and cling, the greater the pain.) Also, this kind of holding on naturally activates and amplifies the striving, willful ego-self. Instead of the gentle release that allows the spirit within to blossom, we're feeding the ego. And the vicious cycle of control, suffering, and pain spirals on.

The irony is this: nowadays we have a wide variety of medications that can be used effectively for palliative and hospice care to alleviate pain and keep the patient comfortable. However, along with the development of these drugs come new and ever more sophisticated and complex treatment options. Life can be prolonged without a cure in sight. In these cases the patient may be kept alive long after a natural death would have occurred.

In response to these interventions, other symptoms and side effects often present themselves: periodic confusion, dyspnea (labored breathing), severe fatigue, incontinence, anorexia, and frequent vomiting, impeding the patient's ability to focus on the emotional and spiritual work of dying. Rather than extending life, the process of dying is being unnaturally elongated. The frustration and anger patients feel at being trapped in this way often produces a kind of "caged rage" that they're reticent to express, as it might upset loved ones. Bottling up these feelings (still another aspect of control) results in not only increased physical pain, but in depression.

When it's clear that there's no way out, this helplessness and desperation intensifies the fear of the Dark Hole. It's at this juncture that many turn to assisted suicide as the only option. In a culture in which there's a powerful unspoken belief that death solves problems (i.e. war, capital punishment, abortion), that there is no value in suffering, and that control is the ultimate goal, it's easy to see why taking one's own life might seem the best option. The ego remains in charge, calling all the shots.

However, this approach robs the patient and loved ones of discovering the fragile beauty of the true, stripped-away self, the enlightenment that can come from experiencing the honing of truth, the clear vision of the meaning of your own life, and clarity of your own center – the place where God dwells. Here, at Signpost 10 on the Path of Suffering, the patient is faced with the greatest mystery of all: Who will I be as my ego-self continues to diminish? Who will I be in my dying? Who will I be on the other side of the grave? Will I be reinvented? Raised up?

It's important to be free enough to stand in the mystery of these questions, the answers revealing themselves when death is allowed to naturally unfold. We cannot be receptive to these revelations when all of our energy is focused on fighting an unwinnable battle - a battle that often trumps loving, life-giving conversations, that blocks expressions of gratitude, preventing us from making meaning of a life and recognizing, at the depth of our souls, that love is the highest ideal of all.

So, there are important choices to be discussed and critical decisions to be made in this quest for freedom, and the sooner they are grappled with, the better. When a patient has done his or her spiritual work, when they have begun to rely more on God, on the true self, and less on the ego-self, these decisions are made much more easily. Instead of attempting to prevent an inevitable death, they look to cooperate with the natural processes that will take place.

DISCUSSING ADVANCE DIRECTIVES

Advance Directives are guidelines and considerations designed to help patients, loved ones, and medical staff make the difficult decisions that walk the fine line between preserving life and ushering in death. What exactly should inform these decisions and help families feel confident that medical choices have been made in the best interest of the patient with respect to the management of physical pain, while meeting the mental, emotional, and spiritual needs of the patient? Having open, honest, loving conversations lays the groundwork for discussing Advance Directives. In the best possible case scenario, the patient should be encouraged to weigh in on these decisions while still able to do so. These are not easy questions to consider and there are few clear answers. Each case is different, as is each patient, each family. All the more reason to grapple with Advance Directives sooner rather than later.

One of my parishioners, Frank, an emergency room nurse in New York City, recently spoke to me about the number of patients he's encountered who find themselves facing end of life care without Advance Directives in place. "Fr. Tom," he said, "people have no idea how much suffering these desperate measures can cause. CPR, chest compressions, intubation, mechanical ventilators, tracheostomies, pacemakers, IV fluids, feeding tubes – all may extend 'life' – but if people had any idea how much physical and emotional distress they can cause in end of life patients..." He shook his head. "Without Advance Directives, a living will, or a health care proxy we're legally bound to do *everything* possible to preserve life. The burden of these decisions often falls to family members who feel obligated to do everything they can to 'save' the life of a loved one, even if it causes or prolongs suffering." Frank looked me straight in the eye. "Fr. Tom," he continued, "you need to tell people to get their ducks in a row before a crisis situation. We all need to take that responsibility in considering the implications of our decisions, or lack of them."

The Catholic Church has looked closely at the ethical questions related to end-of-life issues and has compiled some basic guiding principles to assist those responsible for making these difficult choices. You can find many online resources that lay out the Advance Directives, so rather than repeat them I'm going to highlight some of what I see as the key considerations to take into account.

THE SANCTITY OF LIFE AND END-OF-LIFE CARE

A foundational idea is that medical professionals are pledged to care even when a cure is impossible. It then becomes important to distinguish between *care* and *cure*.

The Church suggests that it is wise to avoid extremes in both directions – burdensome or futile technology used to extend a waning life, or the withdrawal of reasonable care in order to hasten death. The defining factor is whether the protocol of care for the dying is "ordinary or proportionate" as a means of preserving life. The determination used to deem a treatment "proportionate" has to do with weighing the benefit to the patient against any extreme or undue burden or expense for the family.

Another key point has to do with the refusal of ongoing treatment. The Church states:

"When death is imminent and cannot be prevented by the remedies used, it is licit in conscience to decide to renounce treatments that can only yield a precarious and painful prolongation of life...This rejection of a remedy is not to be compared to suicide; it is more justly to be regarded as a simple acceptance of the human condition or a desire to avoid the application of medical techniques that are disproportionate to the value of the anticipated results or, finally, a desire not to put a heavy burden on the family or the community."

This is apropos to Lisa's story – she clearly knew that she did not want to be party to her own painful prolongation of life. The issue with Lisa was that her family was not willing to consider the cessation of treatment. This raises ethical questions about who should make these kinds of determinations. The Church further states:

"In the last analysis, the decision rests with the conscience of the sick person or those who have a right to act in the sick person's name or of the doctors, who must bear in mind the principles of morality and the several aspects of the case..."

The problem is, that often it's easier for a doctor to talk about medical treatment than it is to sensitively address an impending death. But, as the Church states - the decision rests with the conscience of the sick person.

There are a number of ethical questions patients and families should consider. One is whether or not to use pain medication that may inadvertently take the patient from consciousness. If the sole intent is to alleviate pain, and this is the only remaining option, then, in the best interest of the patient, medication such as morphine may be legitimate.

Another vexing decision has to do with the use of artificial nutrition and hydration. Of course, there is a moral obligation to provide the patient with food and water, but what if the patient is unable to eat or drink on their own or by ordinary means with assistance? Should the patient be fed and hydrated by extraordinary means? The Church recommends that when and if artificial nutrition and hydration become the only option, what must be considered is whether or not this would be "excessively burdensome for the patient or would cause significant physical discomfort, for example, resulting from complications in the use of the means employed." Simply put, if death is imminent due to a fatal and progressive disease, forced feeding and hydration can prolong suffering and postpone death, causing additional pain and discomfort. In this situation, the Church assures families that withholding artificial means of delivering nutrition and hydration is often the most ethical thing to do for a loved one.

One personal observation – when families haven't resolved long-standing issues, when goodbyes haven't been said, when conversations that begged to be had have been avoided – these are times when families often experience feelings of guilt and regret when faced with end-of-life decisions. Then, in an unconscious attempt to make it up to the patient, they sometimes go to great lengths to continue to pursue extreme treatment. This is still another reason why loving conversations are a must.

In cases where a patient may lapse into a "persistent vegetative state," making decisions about nutrition and hydration may seem more complicated. The moral compass the Church provides is this: if the patient can be expected to otherwise continue living in this state for an indefinite amount of time, then providing nutrition and hydration becomes our responsibility.

None of these decisions are simple or clear-cut. There are many levels of subjectivity, and some family members may disagree with others' assessment of the situation. Emotions flare, past stories play out, and the water muddies. All the more reason to discuss advance directives, to frankly discuss the range of "what-ifs." Doing so takes tremendous pressure off of loved ones, helps avoid painful and emotionally charged conflicts between family members at a time when they're not in the best frame of mind to make or agree upon critical decisions.

If the family can all get into the same boat and row together in cadence, this can avoid confusion later. Often family members disagree – some want to prolong care, others want to usher in the end, each pointing a finger of blame and guilt at the other. I tell families, "Never rush a decision, and if loved ones are at odds, be kind to one another and invite in the hospice staff, hospital chaplain, priest or minister for guidance.

And, after the fact, try not to look back and rethink it. Assume the integrity of the other, and never judge decisions made in a foxhole."

For more on advance directives see: *Ethical and Religious Directives for Catholic Health Care Services (ERD)*, 5ᵗʰ Ed. , USCCB, 2009; *Euthanasia*, Declaration of the Sacred Congregation for the Doctrine of the Faith (CDF), May 5, 1980; *Nutrition and Hydration: Moral and Pastoral Reflections*, Committee for Pro-Life Activities, National Conference of Catholic Bishops, 1992; *Pope John Paul II on Life-Sustaining Treatment and the Vegetative State (March 20, 2004)*.

PALLIATIVE AND HOSPICE CARE

Both palliative and hospice care offer alternatives to aggressive and ultimately futile treatments, allowing the patient the comfort and dignity often difficult to achieve in a clinical hospital setting. Unfortunately, many people associate palliative and hospice care with "giving up." In fact, it is anything but. Designed to help patients suffering from long-term, generally incurable illnesses, palliative care improves patients' quality of life. And to be clear – palliative care is not limited to those who are terminal. It can also be used to ease the side effects of treatments intended to cure a disease. Palliative care encompasses not only strategies for managing pain, but support in meeting the spiritual, emotional, and practical needs of the patient. It is meant to address the whole person, not just the disease. Included are a combination of strategies for pain relief, counseling, massage, prayer, legal advice, meal preparation, family counseling, even respite support for caregivers – whatever it takes to meet the unique needs of the patient. The goal is to provide the patient with the best possible quality of life for whatever time remains. Most hospitals have a palliative care team made up of specially trained doctors, nurses, social workers, nutritionists, pharmacists, and experts in alternative therapies such as acupuncture and massage.

So what is the difference between palliative care and hospice care? Hospice care is intended for those who have decided to suspend treatment as the hope of a cure is unlikely or impossible. Typically hospice care begins when a patient's life expectancy is estimated to be six months or less. Of course, palliative care is a big part of what hospice offers. The goal is to provide not only the relief of symptoms and pain but the comfort, peace, dignity, and support that the patient and loved ones need. Most patients receive hospice care in their own homes, but there are also facilities devoted to caring for those in the end stages of life. If hospice takes place at home a loved one serves as the primary caregiver and point person, supported by professional hospice staff. The patient's program is designed by an interdisciplinary team (IDT) made up of the patient's personal MD, a hospice specialist, nurses, a pharmacologist, nutritionist, counselors, therapists, social workers, a priest or minister, a case manager, as well as trained volunteers. Home Health Aids can be assigned to help with personal care-taking such as bathing and toileting. The team collaborates on an individualized plan to meet the unique needs of each family, and once in place, arranges regular visits to reassess the situation and adjust the plan as necessary. Hospice support is available 24 hours a day, every day. Your medical team, hospital social worker, or pastoral care staff can suggest when hospice care is appropriate and provide information on the best way to initiate it.

THE PATH TO CLOSURE

Dealing with the practical realities of an impending death will help you to check the baggage you carry with you on this final journey. Lightening your load by telling your stories, simplifying your lifestyle, getting your house in order, making decisions in regard to advance directives, palliative care, and hospice – all of this clears the way so that the remainder of the path can lead you to a place of gentle, loving closure. Relinquishing control, putting the ego self in the back seat creates a space for the spirit self to begin to drive the car. When the spirit self leads, the focus becomes a thrust toward loving others unconditionally, and letting yourself be vulnerable enough to graciously accept the love and care of others, no matter how limited or flawed that human love may be. Instead of feeling like the road to death, you begin to understand that you're really continuing the journey of the soul. Bolstered by God's strength, God's courage, and God's wisdom, strive to do little things with great love, offer affirmation and affection whenever possible, and then, begin to say your goodbyes.

CHAPTER 29

Affirmation, Affection, Gratitude, and Goodbyes

"Father, they are your gift to me. I wish that where I am they also may be with me, that they may see my glory that you gave me, because you loved me before the foundation of the world. Righteous Father, the world also does not know you, but I know you, and they know that you sent me. I made known to them your name and I will make it known, that the love with which you loved me may be in them and I in them."

-- JOHN 17:24-26

IN HIS FINAL hours, Jesus prayed this prayer within earshot of his disciples. While it is intercessory in nature, the fact that Jesus offered it publicly suggests that he was trying to communicate a final message of love and truth to those closest to him. As his last minutes drew ever nearer, Jesus fervently imparted this final discourse.

For anyone on the Path of Suffering, approaching his or her own death, there is much to learn from Jesus' example. After talking with so many people on the Path of Suffering, I believe that Jesus' sentiments are the same ones we'd all like to share with those we love, if we only knew how. At funeral masses I always tell families to listen carefully to this passage – that it is, indeed, what the deceased wants them to understand. Listen to it again, gently reframed, from the point of view of someone you love in his or her final days, when values and priorities become crystal clear:

Father, my family and friends have been your gifts to me. I wish that where I am they also may be with me, so that they may see my glory that you gave me, because you loved me before the foundation of the world. Dearest Father, the world also does not know you, but I now know you, and my family and friends will know that you sent me. I made known to those I love your name and I will make it known, that the love with which you loved me may be in them and I in them. " –John 17:26.

What a legacy to leave. What a message of hope – in the midst of one's suffering, a testament to the indwelling of God. An affirmation of the fact that, in death, our loved one becomes one with God, and since God dwells within each of us, then our loved one also will dwell within *us*. Perfect oneness. Unity. Communion.

How difficult it must have been for Jesus to reach beyond his own grief and pain in order to make this point. You might be thinking how difficult it would be for you, me, or any of us, in our own hour of suffering. How can we extend this kind of affirmation and affection, gratitude, and goodbye, when our day comes?

Before answering, let's reflect for a moment on what I've referred to as Signpost 10 along the Path of Suffering: Who am I Becoming? Perhaps, of all the signposts, #10 is the most significant. It addresses the issue we most naturally want to avoid, and that is *change*. Throughout this book, we've become more aware of our own defense mechanisms, the influence of our culture, the true nature of God, the wounds of our lives and their effects, dynamics of family, and communication. In attempting to embrace new ways of thinking, engaging in spiritual practices, striving mindfully to do little things with great love, conversion gradually occurs. Hopefully it has. Accepting all of these changes requires a radical dying to self, a letting go of all assumptions, a surrender of the ego self. Thus, it naturally conjures the question, "Who am I becoming? " a question those along the Path of Suffering have to ask time and time again. The ego self diminishes, and the spirit self more fully emerges, making the kind of heart-felt message Jesus shared all the more possible.

How can we gauge the extent to which our fulcrum has shifted?

The answer is, by the fruit we bear. By the nature of our loving. By our willingness to be vulnerable. As the ego self diminishes we have less of a need to make sense of everything, to continually ask "why." We begin to rely more on God than on self, and when we extend ourselves in love we have no expectations of return. As the fulcrum shifts we experience a freedom from past hurts, the ability and willingness to embrace those with whom we've struggled. We can begin to see everything in the past as gift, all those who hurt us or let us down as instruments for learning acceptance and compassion. We learn to listen with ears of sensitivity and kindness, recognizing and healing the wounds driving the hurtful, insensitive words. This time can also be an amazing opportunity to allow yourself to be completely open and vulnerable to receive the gifts of affection, care, and love offered by others and bathe yourself in it, and also to reassure them that you'll be all right, that they don't need to feel any regret, guilt, or any sense of over-responsibility because you're secure in God's care and promise. You're past the point of hanging on to expectations, of making demands. Those behaviors are laid down with the ego self. Now, the fulcrum is tipped in the other direction. Instead of trying to make deals with God, we trust God as being steadfastly loving and merciful. We know we have little strength on our own, and we acknowledge that whatever strength and courage we have is born of God. We're comfortable detaching from our titles, positions, accomplishments, and possessions. Our loneliness becomes solitude. Inner stillness and peace have taken the place of anxiety and fear. We gradually come to see that we're part of a much bigger story, and experience solidarity and oneness with all that is.

As I write this, however, I want to be clear. The fulcrum moves, day-to-day, hour-to-hour. I'm not suggesting that *any* of us experience this kind of transformation perfectly – not even close. We backslide and we regress because we're human. But think back to the beginning of this journey. Ask yourself who you were then, and who you are now. Are you freer to love? Freer to forgive? More empathetic and understanding

315

than you were before? Being emptied creates room for this gradual transformation. And transformation is a *process.*

One more point – if you or a loved one haven't undergone this change – perhaps your life story has held you prisoner longer, producing deeper wounds that require more time to heal – there's no need to fear the human "finish line." Remember the Sacred Spiral in chapter 19? The transformative work left uncompleted here is continued beyond the grave. There is hope for each and every one of us. As Jesus said in John 18:9, *"I have not lost one of whom you have given me."*

WHAT WILL YOUR FINAL DISCOURSE BE?

Once the practicalities of putting your house in order and making critical decisions about your care are behind you, you're free to do the most important work of all – to express your deepest sentiments to those you love. Now is the time to further focus this outward movement, to intensify your loving through expressions of affirmation, affection, and gratitude as you strive to say your goodbyes.

I can't tell you how often I've witnessed the dying fight the disease to the last moment, lapse into what I call the "red zone" of coma or unconsciousness without ever having taken the opportunity to say "Thank you," "This is what you've meant to me," "Forgive me," "Here is what life has taught me." "This is what I know to be true." "Here is what I know about God." Leaving these words unsaid makes the mourning process so much more difficult for those left behind.

On the other hand, I've had the privilege of witnessing and sometimes facilitating the kinds of loving conversations that change the experience of death for both the patient and his or her loved ones. I can't stress enough how important it is to do this work in the "green zone," sooner rather than later. This is when I usually say to them, "It's time. You've got work to do!" How delighted the dying are to embrace "good work," to mark their impending death with freedom, light, and love!

Here are some stories of real, ordinary people who, in their dying, loved in extraordinary ways. It wasn't easy, but their willingness to let go, to move out of their comfort zones in the interest of others, was nothing short of life changing.

MILLIE'S STORY

Diane's mother Millie was in her eighties and had always enjoyed good health. But a series of cardiac events sent her into the hospital where she suffered congestive heart failure. She grew weaker by the day, the stress on her heart increasing. Diane called me to come to the hospital. I gave Millie *viaticum*, or food for the journey (part of what we Catholics used to refer to as the "last rites"). We talked about the "work of dying as the working of loving." I told her to individually affirm and appreciate the important people in her life. Millie, a southern girl who grew up in Louisiana, took to the idea of demonstrating her love in an intensive way like a fish to water. She realized that her time was limited and she didn't waste a minute. She was conscious and alert, but she knew at the core of her being that her life was coming to an end.

One by one she called her children, grandchildren, and other family members into her room, invited them to sit beside her bed. She took their hands and described to each of them the gift they'd specifically been to her, and told them how much she loved them. She also professed the faith that had sustained her through the years, and how she was not afraid to die. She reassured each of them, attesting to the power of God in her life.

When she died, of course everyone was sad, but there was a lingering sense of the peace, joy, and love that became her legacy. To this day when Diane speaks about her mother's final days it's with a sense of awe and gratitude.

CHARLIE'S STORY

Charlie had been a faithful parishioner, attending Eucharist every Sunday with his wife Clare. Before every mass my habit is to circulate through the church, greeting and touching base with the congregation. It helps me connect with parishioners, gauge the climate, and make myself available to them. This is how I noticed that of late, Charlie's wife Clare had been coming alone. When I asked Clare where Charlie was, she teared up. "He has cancer," she said. "It's really serious."

I asked Clare if I could come and bring Charlie communion, and she enthusiastically agreed. Later that day I stopped by for a visit and Charlie and I talked. Charlie knew his cancer was stage 4, and clearly understood that a cure or even a remission was not a possibility. Being a man of faith, he told me he wasn't afraid, just sad.

"Charlie," I said, "you have work to do. The most important work of your life."

Interestingly, while Charlie wasn't afraid of dying, he was extremely uncomfortable expressing his emotions. "Charlie's one who doesn't like talking about that kind of thing," Clare said. "My man of few words..."

"Well," I said to Charlie, "I did tell you there was work to do. It isn't meant to be easy! Now, let's go!"

"I'll leave you two," Clare said, and slipped out of the room. I could feel her discomfort and disappointment at his seeming inability to express himself in this way.

"Charlie...do you love your wife? "

"Of course I love my wife!"

"Have you told her? "

"She knows I love her. I was a good husband."

"This isn't a time to be cheap with words. Tell her! And your daughter. This is a unique opportunity to tell each of them the gift they've been to you. What you cherish about them. Thank them. Explain to them what life's taught you. Tell them your hopes for them. And most important, give them a witness to your faith. A faith so strong that you're not afraid to die! Now come on! Get going!"

In the weeks that followed Charlie indeed did his "assignment." And once he started, this man of few words opened up, making up for lost time. By the time he went to hospice, he had told his wife and daughter specifically what gifts they'd been, how they were the center of his world, and that his courage - especially the particular courage it took for him to find the words he found so difficult to say - was rooted in God.

I visited him a day or so before he died. Clare and their daughter Becky followed me into the hallway, embraced me, and tearfully thanked me for what I'd done for Charlie. The intimacy shared through his vulnerability was a rare and precious thing – a gift they could never have imagined receiving in the midst of this great loss.

My Mom's Story

Throughout her life my mother was plagued by fears and anxieties. She was a classic hypochondriac, worrying unnecessarily about imagined ailments. At age 82 she was diagnosed with colon cancer that had spread to the liver. Never a warm and fuzzy type, unsentimental and earthy, my mother had a quick wit and sometimes a sharp tongue. So you can imagine our surprise when in the final stages of liver cancer she shared something profound with several of her granddaughters gathered around her, on her favorite couch. The disease had stolen her edge, and mostly she sat quietly, seemingly fading away.

But this visit was different. As her granddaughters gently massaged her hands, Granny suddenly became animated, and the girls felt an unusual energy in the room. Granny stared off in the distance and said, "Do you see him? "

"See who, Granny? "

My mother continued, "Have you told him you love him? "

The cousins exchanged a glance, thinking she was teasing. "Who Granny? We don't have any boyfriends."

My mother, still intent and very much focused said, "The change is coming, and I'm not afraid." Given who she was, this was a surprising statement. She went on, "I'm just sad because I'll be leaving you."

They all believed it was Jesus she was seeing, and suddenly felt a little afraid at this revelation, so much so that they ran into the other room to get their mothers. When they returned Granny was calm and peaceful.

Her witness left a deep impression on the teens. If Granny wasn't afraid, then what was there to fear?

PHIL'S STORY

We met Phil in Chapter 17. After he returned from Sloan to die at home, he was confined to bed, balloons on his legs to help control the massive swelling. One day his wife Sandy was tending to his needs, bending over beside his bed, when she felt a pinch on her backside. She straightened up and turned. There was Phil, a crooked smile playing on his lips. Despite his compromised body, she saw the shadow of the mischievous, affectionate "bad boy" she'd fallen in love with. Sandy laid down beside him, and Phil nestled his head in the crook of her neck. Sandy stroked his hair, and they spoke of how much they loved one another, how precious their shared life had been. Both of them were totally vulnerable, realizing that a moment like this might not occur again. Phil died several days later. It was one of the most intimate and profound experiences Sandy has ever had – one that she cherishes.

MY FATHER'S STORY

Both of my parents, being of Irish heritage and a certain generation, found it difficult under even the best of circumstances to say, "I love you." They preferred to show their love through gestures, usually involving food (which is probably why I've struggled with my weight for years.) So when my father was dying, and confined to a nursing home, I knew it was time to help usher in the words my sisters and I longed to hear.

Sometimes we need to become the facilitator in these situations. A couple of my sisters felt that asking my dad to say, "I love you," somehow negated the sincerity of it. I, however, have never felt that way. To me, it's foolish to sit and wait for a "golden nugget" that isn't likely to be given without encouragement. Here's how this played out in my family.

"Big T" (as we affectionately called him) was winding down. We all knew that it was only a matter of a couple of months before he died, but he steadfastly avoided any words of affirmation or affection. Since his love had always been expressed through "doing" for us rather than by "telling" us his feelings, he felt as though his opportunities to show his love were long past.

During one visit I told him, "Dad, you have to extend your repertoire. You need to tell people that you love them. Me, your daughters, your grandchildren."

"It's not what you say to people, Tommy, it's what you *do* for them. I know plenty of people who say 'I love you' and they're full of crap."

I thought about this. Sure, sometimes it was true. But it was also true that others who said it, *did* mean it. And some who could say it, just couldn't get it together to show it.

I thought back to when my sister Maureen had died. How, even at her deathbed my dad couldn't tell her he loved her. He felt badly about it afterward, but he just couldn't do it. All these needless regrets...

"I know you missed your chance with Maureen. And your days of 'doing' for us are over. So, now it's time to use words."

Big T grimaced and waved his hand weakly at me.

Because I knew, deep down, that he loved me I pressed on. "Dad, so you're telling me none of us needs to hear that we're loved? "

He stubbornly shook his head.

I walked over to his bulletin board where a collection of cards from his children and grandchildren hung. I took my pen out and pretended to cross out the words of love they'd all written to him.

My father's blue eyes flashed. "Tommy, stop it! You're crazy!"

"Oh," I said playfully. "So you DO crave those words!" I kissed him on top of his headful of curly white hair and turned to go. "Think about it, Dad," I said with a smile. "I'll be back!"

A couple of days later I made a return visit. "So, Dad, are you ready to tell me how much you love me? "

He shook his head as if I was something to be tolerated, but I saw the smile he was trying to hide.

"Try it..." I urged. "Say Tommy, I love you. Come on..."

Big T pressed his lips together. Rolled his eyes.

"Come on, Dad, repeat it. Tommy, I love you!"

Finally he stuck out his chin and said, "Tommy I love you!" It was a little like wringing a drop of water from a washcloth. Before I could respond he added, "Now turn around, bend over, and I'll kiss your ass." He grinned like the cat that swallowed the canary.

"Gee, Dad, you couldn't be vulnerable for one minute!" I teased. We both had a good laugh. But he'd said it.

After that, whenever I left he told me he loved me. I would thank him and tell him I loved him too. It became our special ritual every time I saw him until the day he died.

It also required gentle persistence, and a willingness to be vulnerable in asking. A sense of humor was also a must. But it was worth it. Not long afterward he wrote the following note and had it sent to all of his children and grandchildren:

Thank you for your cards and communications to me. I am happy to receive them, especially from my grandchildren. I enjoy reading about the daily comings and goings of their lives. I am doing my best to enjoy the type of life I have left to spend. I have been very fortunate over the years in more ways than one. I keep telling myself, "Tommy, you are alive, it triumphs over everything else. At my age, everything is small stuff.

Old age in a nursing home is not for wimps. I will be here until the time comes. You have to take a lot of wrapping and rewrapping every day. I do try to be cheerful during your visits. Keep me in your prayers. I spend a lot of my spare time praying for you. May your life be as blessed as my life has.

Love, Poppa

My dad isn't the only one I know who expressed heartfelt feelings in writing. One parishioner dictated personal notes for loved ones to a hospice volunteer. While not as personal as exchanging words and touch, face-to-face, the thought and care expressed in a tangible way touched many hearts. These notes were read and reread, tucked between the pages of a family Bible, or slipped into a nightstand drawer where they were readily accessible on days when the recipients needed to be reminded that they were loved, that God is present even in darkness, and that life, despite its challenges, is beautiful. Another parishioner wrote a letter to be read at her funeral, her sentiments stretching beyond the grave – a powerful account of what life had taught her, how God had sustained her, along with tender words of gratitude and love. Significant, loving words shared at any time make an impression, but perhaps none are as impactful as those expressed in the shadow of death.

Similarly, I've worked with parents who were terminally ill, who felt a deep need to express themselves to their children, who, at the time, lacked the maturity to understand the depth of feelings that needed to be expressed. Over a period of months, they recorded videos in which they spoke directly to their children. Words of love came freely, and I've witnessed them record footage to be played at future milestones, carrying messages appropriate to the ages of children at that time. Words of wisdom and love for first communion, graduation, weddings, the birth of a child, reaching across time and space. Not only would these videos be treasured through the years, but they provided a sense of accomplishment and closure for the patient.

REASSURANCE

The first syllable of the word "farewell" comes from an old English word meaning 'to journey.' Now-a-days the word "fare" (as in faring well) means 'to manage.' Saying farewell, therefore, suggests that as loved ones part, each desires that the other may journey well - and manage well. This also applies to the person moving toward an impending death and beyond, as well as family and friends who must continue on after the end of their loved one's earthly life.

Often the terminally ill patient will hang on longer than is reasonable, worrying about how loved ones will fare in the wake of his/her death. This is another instance where sharing words of affirmation, affection, gratitude and goodbye are important. Sometimes these loving words spoken by family and friends offer the support one needs to let go and move on to the next phase. Over and over again I've witnessed family members finally telling a loved one, "It's okay...we'll be fine. We know how tired you are. It's all right to go. We love you so much..." Remarkably, after these reassuring words, the patient often settles down and, within hours, passes peacefully. Clearly, words have power.

Let's go back for a moment and reflect on the reframing of the words of Jesus that we presented at the beginning of this chapter...

> *Father, my family and friends have been your gifts to me. I wish that where I am they also may be with me, so that they may see my glory that you gave me, because you loved me before the foundation of the world. Dearest Father, the world also does not know you, but I know you, and my family and friends will know that you sent me. I made known to those I love your name and I will make it known, that the love with which you loved me may be in them and I in them.*

Sharing similar words of love with family and friends in the face of impending death is a gift that continues to open the door to transformation, not only for the person about to cross over, but for the recipients of these sentiments.

Some people in these situations, however, take these efforts even further along in the manner of Jesus' example. In addition to exchanging words of love, they bare not only their hearts, but the depth of their souls to the other. As the ego self diminishes, the spirit self emerges with greater clarity. God's spirit spills over, resulting in an intimate witness that has the power to transform others. These kinds of exchanges in the eleventh hour of life can help both parties see more clearly who they are in God, bringing their relationship to a level of intimacy they could previously not have imagined.

CHAPTER 30

Death is at the Door

ALL RITES OF passage involve struggle and loss. The pilgrim traveler must die to the familiar, and what will be birthed from this isn't yet apparent. Actual death, unlike other rites of passage such as marriage, is the most profound, because the reality on the other side cannot, by its very nature, be known.

Therefore, the process of dying is steeped in mystery. Our dying time is cut from the ordinary, in a space undefined by the natural rhythms of life. Normal routines, schedules, responsibilities fall away for everyone involved – for the person in the bed as well as the loved ones in vigil around the bed. In this way, the dying days, hours, and minutes are sacred – time set apart for a deeper encounter with God. The time seems endless, yet fleeting. There is an urge to hold on and an impulse to let go. There is the futile medical accouterment juxtaposed against a surreal sense of hovering at a threshold; of a momentous event about to occur characterized by something as subtle as a final exhalation.

Father Richard Rohr describes this as follows: "*Limen* is the Latin word for threshold. A 'liminal space' is the crucial in-between time – when everything actually happens and yet nothing appears to be happening. It is the waiting period when the cake bakes, the movement is made, the transformation takes place."

The Irish call these paradoxical experiences "thin spaces," A thin space can be defined as a fault or fissure between heaven and earth, allowing those with the eyes to see to experience God in a unique moment of clarity. Jesus explained this to Martha at the death of her brother Lazarus, who had died in Jesus' absence. Jesus said to Martha, *"If you believe, you will see the glory of God."* (John 11:40)

And so can we. Through eyes of faith we can stand in the liminal space at the edge of death and experience the presence of God in our loved one who is dying, and vice versa. We can tap into the palpable sense of the sacred, into the threshold between heaven and earth. We can commune with our loved one in ways that are more profound than words, more meaningful than memories, more powerful than impending loss or sadness.

As in any sacred experience, we can better facilitate this in a number of ways through rites and rituals that are rich in symbolism. What can we do to ensure that all involved enter fully into this sacred space and time?

SIGNS THAT DEATH APPROACHES

There is a point at which a person realizes that he or she is no longer looking to a future in which they're going to die, but that the future is upon them. This is the difference between "going to die" and the realization that "I am dying." As loved ones gather around the bed, there are certain signs that death is close at hand. These symptoms and behaviors may start gradually, months or weeks before, and intensify with time. Throughout a terminal illness, the patient's energy level and physical strength wane. As this happens, the patient may withdraw from others. Experience an aversion to eating. Eventually the patient may have difficulty swallowing and begin to avoid solid food. It's important for loved ones to respect this, to resist the inclination to urge them to eat. When my mother was dying my father would constantly bring her food. "Come on, you have to eat," he'd say. According to him, if she ate she'd regain her strength. But, she wasn't hungry. Her body no longer needed nutrition. Forcing it only made her more uncomfortable.

More and more hours are spent sleeping, sometimes fitfully. The patient may lapse in and out of consciousness, experience periods of restlessness and confusion. In the final hours the patient may gradually lose control of all body functions. Their temperature will drop, and as circulation decreases the extremities may become cold and pale.

Breathing patterns change as death is close at hand. Exhalation breaths become longer than inhalations. Breathing may become erratic and labored, then may increase in frequency, engaging the entire rib cage. Often, breathing may cease for up to ten or more seconds before the next inhalation. This can happen for days or, in some cases, even for weeks. Finally, a rattling sound may occur with each breath.

Many times there is what I call a brief "last hurrah," in which the patient seems to dramatically improve, become alert and animated, engaging in a lucid way with loved ones. When this happens it's a rare opportunity to share some last precious moments in an active, conscious way.

The final signs that death is imminent include a fixed stare, dilated pupils, the color draining from the lips, hands and feet, replaced by a gray or bluish tone. The patient no longer responds to stimuli, and breathing eventually ceases.

Being sensitive to these signs, providing gentle affirmation and loving responsiveness is key. Hospice workers are experienced at reading these signs and will assist loved ones in the best and most timely ways to offer comfort and support.

Pastoral Care for the Dying

It's important, during this sacred transition time, to strike the right balance – to assist, but not interfere, to support, but not hinder. Compassionately standing beside the loved one, as a peaceful presence, reassuring them of the sacredness of this most intimate of times makes it easier for the dying to let go and pass through the threshold more easily. There are a number of ways to establish an environment of peaceful calm – using powerful symbols of faith, putting together an ancestral shrine, playing soothing music, administering tender massage or touch, "feeding" the person the sacred word, and, when the patient is just too ill to pray, to become their prayer. Throughout all of this, seeing, acknowledging, and loving God within the other establishes a deep communion. Let's look at each of these rituals.

DISPLAY THE CRUCIFIX

I always suggest that Christian families display a crucifix in the room within the view of the patient. The cross itself is a symbol of a liminal space – the horizontal axis connecting us one to another, intersecting the vertical axis reaching heaven to earth. The symbol of Christ on the Cross is a vivid reminder that, as we approach our deaths, we too are "nailed to our suffering." At a certain point, there is nothing to do but hang there in it. Surrender to it.

Suffering to death is universal human reality, which Jesus experienced first-hand. We realize that we worship a God who understands our suffering, who walked this path ahead of us. I ask the dying to reflect on the crucifix and to repeat the words Jesus proclaimed from the cross, *"Into your hands I commend my spirit..."* When we "commend our spirit," we surrender, in faith, to who we are becoming through this death. We begin to cross the threshold, to make the transition. This brings new meaning and relevance to the memorial acclamation we recite at mass: *Save us, Savior of the world, for by your cross and resurrection you have set us free.* This can be translated into a prayer for the dying, substituting their name, as follows: *Save (name), Savior of the world, for by your cross and resurrection, you have set (him/her) free.* The cross inextricably ties together death with resurrection – the two cannot be separated. Gazing on the cross with this in mind brings both comfort and hope.

ANCESTRAL SHRINES

Setting up a "shrine" of photographs and mementos of deceased relatives and friends who most loved the patient, along with pictures of favorite saints is a reminder that they are within you and will help you make this cross over from death to new life. Of course, it's not as though these deceased loved ones suddenly appear to usher the patient to heaven – in fact they're already one with God, and therefore already dwelling within the patient. Instead, the shrine helps the patient open her or himself more fully to this indwelling, to feel supported as a sojourner, and to be comforted by the fact that these loved ones have walked this path. Most importantly, the patient realizes that he/she isn't making this passing alone. The shrine is really a celebration of the "communion of saints" and a reminder of the oneness that reaches across the grave.

I always tell patients that as they surrender in love, their awareness of the indwelling – of God and with all who have passed on before them - increases. As the intuitive liminal floodgate slowly opens, this awareness grows and begins to pulsate – it is a movement of deep love and sure knowing.

EXPERIENCING GOD'S AFFECTION

Soft, expressive music, a tender massage, a view of the glory of nature, a warm breeze against the face, sun on the shoulders – all are expressions of God's affection. At the Connecticut Hospice in Branford, CT, windows open to broad vistas of Long Island Sound. There are paths and benches, gazebos and shade trees that patients and families can experience together. This kind of gentle sensory stimulation can root the patient strongly in the present, awakening a deeper awareness of God's presence and a profound feeling of being one with all that is. I recently went with my friend to visit his mother in a nursing home, and we found her sitting in the atrium, the sun kissing her face. She seemed so peaceful, almost heavenly. I turned and said to her son, *"Look - your mom is being embraced by her God."*

These experiences all focus on *being* rather than on *doing.* The patient becomes the recipient of sensory input that conveys love and care, with no expectation to have to return it. Sitting beside the patient, tenderly stroking his or her hand, swabbing their lips, bringing a source of music, a scented candle, a bouquet of wildflowers, turning the bed toward a window as the sun beams in... Being able to "be" in this way allows the patient to rest in the hands and heart of God.

FEEDING THE PATIENT THE SACRED WORD

As patients inch closer to death, the scriptures take on new meaning and suddenly explode with relevance:

- *Come to me, all you who labor and are burdened, and I will give you rest. Take my yoke upon you and learn from me, for I am meek and humble of heart; and you will find rest for yourselves. For my yoke is easy, and my burden light. –Matthew 11:28-29.*
- *The Lord is my shepherd; there is nothing I lack. In green pastures he makes me lie down; to still waters he leads me; he restores my soul. – Psalm 23:1-3*
- *Do not let your hearts be troubled. You have faith in God; have faith also in me. In my Father's house there are many dwelling places. If there were not, would I have told you that I am going to prepare a place for you? And if I go and prepare a place for you, I will come back again and take you to myself, so that where I am you also may be. – John 14:1-3*
- *Amen, amen, I say to you, unless a grain of wheat falls to the ground and dies, it remains just a grain of wheat; but if it dies, it produces much fruit. – John 12:24*
- *Jesus said to the crowd: This is the will of the one who sent me that I should not lose anything of what he gave me, but that I should raise it on the last day. For this is the will of my father, that everyone who sees the Son and believes in him may have eternal life, and I shall raise him on the last day. – John 6:39-40*

Taking a line or two from scripture, and reading it to the patient is a balm for the soul, providing comfort and consolation. We often forget that not only is Christ present in the bread and the wine, but in the Word proclaimed. Even as patients slip in and out of consciousness, when they can no longer eat or drink, they can be fed and nourished on God's word. As Jesus said in Matthew 4:4: *Man does not live on bread alone, but on every word that comes from the heart of God.*

Alternately, short lines of scripture can be written on large index cards and taped to the wall near the bed. As long as patients are conscious, this can provide solace during times when they might feel alone.

Here are some short texts that can be used for this purpose, a line at a time, or repeated as a mantra:

- *Who can separate us from the love of Christ? Romans 8:35*
- *Whether we live or die, we are the Lord's. Romans 14:8*
- *We have an everlasting home in heaven. 2 Corinthians 5:1*
- *We shall be with the Lord for ever. 1 Thessalonians 4:17*
- *We have passed from death to life because we love each other. 1 John 3:14*
- *The Lord is my light and my salvation. Psalm 27:1*
- *My soul thirsts for the living God. Psalm 42:3*
- *Though I walk in the shadow of death, I will fear no evil, for you are with me. Psalm 23:4*

BECOMING THE PATIENT'S PRAYER

As death approaches it sometimes becomes impossible for the patient to articulate or even focus on prayer. At these times a real gift is to "become the prayer" of the patient, praying on her or his behalf. Anyone can become a proxy in prayer – a loved one, neighbor, or a church community. The prayers of others create a positive "energy field of love" that can be experienced by the patient, that can open them to the God within. These prayers can be improvised aloud or formally recited in the presence of the patient, or can be prayed in silence or in private on the patient's behalf. Perhaps the patient had a particular favorite prayer or devotion, such as the recitation of the rosary – if so, this can be offered for him/her in love.

THE SUPPORT OF A COMMUNITY OF FAITH

When the patient is in the dying process, the faith community can be approached in order to become a companion on this most sacred journey. There are a number of ways that a community of faith can offer support at this challenging time:

- **Be Remembered in Prayer:**

A loved one can ask for the patient to be remembered in their prayers and have his/her name added to the church prayer list. When a faith community lifts someone up in prayer, it is an act of love that can deepen the faith of everyone involved.

- **Blessing One Another**

People often misunderstand the meaning of the word blessing, limiting it to the idea of God doing something a little extra. *Being blessed is really the ability to recognize the working of God in our lives.* We so often forget God in the equation of both the good and challenging times, or we thank God for the good and blame God for the bad. But God never causes the ups and downs - God provides us with the grace to be thankful for the good and the strength to withstand what is difficult. Being blessed also allows us to transform the challenges into life-giving experiences. Giving or receiving a blessing is an intention to have our eyes opened in faith. So, blessing one another is a gift that all involved can come to cherish. There's no one right way to do it. You can make the sign of the cross on one another's forehead and say, *"God loves you and I love you, too."* Or, *"The Lord is with you."* You might also share this prayer: *"May we see the working of God's love manifested in us as we love and care for each other."* Pause for a moment, in silence, with an open heart. In the quiet, thank God for being an instrument of His love through the other.

When leaving, you can exchange another blessing: *"May you know the peace of God, today and in your tomorrows."*

The Celebration of *Viaticum* for the Dying

When it is determined that a patient will likely pass away in less than a week's time they may receive the sacrament of Viaticum. "Viaticum" is often referred to as "food for the journey," preparing the recipient for the transition from death to new life with God. I always try to visit patients in the "green or yellow zones" while they're still conscious and can swallow. This sacrament is accompanied by a special ritual that includes sprinkling with holy water to remind them of their baptism, a penance rite and apostolic pardon, scripture readings, and a renewal of baptismal promises, all of which emphasize God's mercy, lightening the earthly load, and helping prepare the person for their "crossing over."

PRAYER AFTER DEATH

When a loved one has died, gather together around the bed in sacred silence, recognizing that you are standing at the threshold, on holy ground. The family is encouraged to open their hearts to this grace-filled moment, making an act of faith that their loved one, in experiencing death as Jesus did, will therefore also share in his resurrection. You may also pray as the father who brought his son to Jesus for healing prayed: *Lord, I believe. Help me in my unbelief.*

– Mark 9:24.

One person may lead the following prayer – a family member, friend, or a minister - and the others can pray along by repeating each phrase, or one person may pray it on the family's behalf.

Loving and merciful God we entrust your beloved son/daughter to your mercy. You loved him/her greatly in this life: now that he/she is freed from all its care, give him/her happiness and peace forever. The old order has passed away: welcome him/her into paradise where there will be no more sorrow, no more weeping or pain, but only peace and joy with Jesus, your Son, and the Holy Spirit for ever and ever. Amen.

Then pray the Our Father and Hail Mary together and mark the deceased with the sign of the cross, saying: *Christ has died, Christ has risen. Dearest Lord, thank you for your gift of resurrection for _____.*

REVERENCING THE BODY BY WASHING IT

A beautiful and intimate final act of loving care involves washing the body of the deceased to prepare it for burial. When Barbara's mother died, the nurse gently invited Barbara to participate as much or as little as she liked. Here is Barbara's journal entry, outlining this last physical encounter with her mother.

Nurse Jennifer runs the water until it's warm – how strange, I think, to worry about the temperature. She fills and carries a pink tub and white washcloth over to the bed. The basin and the towel, I think, the Holy Thursday ritual. Something inside of me reverberates and moves me deeply. Oh, how that Jesus really knew what he was doing…

Jennifer begins by touching the cloth in the water and dabbing around my mother's eyes. "I'll do it," I say, and she hands me the cloth. I dip and wipe, gently, tentatively. Her face, her neck. We unsnap the johnnie coat and fold it away. My mother, exposed, her breasts still full, her skin really lovely except for the blotched bruises on her arms from the blood thinners and IV's. A narrow white bandage down the middle of her abdomen. So vulnerable, these fresh stiches, so futile. She lays exposed, all of her, more of her than I'd felt comfortable seeing in these past years, too much familiarity with bodily functions that I'd prefer would have been private. But today, it feels like a sacrament, this exposure an intimacy we hadn't been able to share in life. And her feet. The thick, yellowed nails sculpted by some nursing home doctor – she was always so ashamed of her feet. I wash them, rub lotion all over her, head to toe – an anointing, like Mary Magdalene with the perfumed nard. And I think, sadly and with a tinge of guilt, how it is easier to minister to her in death than it was in life. I ask Jennifer if I can have a moment alone with her.

"Of course." She slips out of the room without a sound. It is just my mother and me. I talk, at first feeling awkward, but then the words flow…

"I'm sorry Mom, I couldn't love you better… We both did the best we could, though, didn't we? Mostly I'm sorry you didn't embrace and enjoy

this world more, that you couldn't feel what I feel as I move through it. That you couldn't realize some kind of dream, aspiration. But I want to thank you for doing for me everything you could. For praying me into existence. For being proud of me. I hope you're free now, and whole. I love you." I bend over her for a couple of more moments, then I leave.

Barbara's experience, after many years of a somewhat negative and strained relationship with her mother, really captures the way that their relationship had already begun to heal. As her mother passed from the woundedness of life into the unconditional love, mercy, and healing of God, the dynamic shifted. Barbara, in extending herself beyond her comfort zone, in her own vulnerability, was able to sense the "whole-making" that God extends to us as we die in His arms.

CHAPTER 31

From Death to New Life

CELEBRATING FUNERAL RITES AND RITUALS

IN THE BOOK "The Death of a Christian: The Order of Christian Funerals," by Reverend Richard Rutherford, CSC, he writes,

"Funeral ritual belongs to the very heritage of the human community. Speaking with the authority of scholarly consensus, the anthropologist Margaret Mead once said, 'I know of no people for whom the fact of death is not critical, and who have no ritual by which to deal with it.'"

More and more these days, I hear families explain that there will be no service, or that they've decided to forgo the funeral mass in favor of a short graveside or funeral home prayer. They mention "not wanting to put the family through it." Or a sense of "just wanting to get it over with." Other times, the terminal patient may insist that he or she doesn't want any kind of service. The reasons for this vary. It could be the expense, or it could be a continuation of a life-long pattern of being unable to accept the love and care of others. Whatever the reason, not having a service robs loved ones of the chance to enter into the mystery in a healing way. Marking this rite of passage is not important for the deceased, who is *already* safely in the hand of God! Without marking this extremely significant event, those left behind are denied the opportunity to face their own mortality, vulnerability, and losses and to see death through the lens of faith and hope.

In my 46 years of ministry I've seen, time and again, the ways that mishandling this major rite of passage can result in generational wounds that rarely fully heal. Sacred closure is *that* important.

This is why I so strongly believe in the importance of celebrating life and reverencing death through the three movements of the funeral ritual, in a place and time separated from the ordinary:

THE VIGIL TIME, THE FUNERAL SERVICE, AND THE COMMITTAL/BURIAL

What we often fail to realize is that each of these three movements corresponds to the respective phases of the Journey of the Soul, rooting the deceased's story – yesterday, today, and tomorrow - firmly in God. If done well (rather than condensing them all into one brief service) the three movements provide an opportunity for the bereaved to reflect on and process the significance of the deceased's life and death, and to better answer the question, "Where has God been in this? And where is God in *my* life?" When the time and energy is taken to approach the mystery in this way, those left behind will invariably leave the graveside more free, more secure in God's love and care, with a sense of hope and deeper faith.

The purpose of funeral rites, as I have always understood it, is perfectly summed up by Cardinal Blase Cupich in a memorial given at an evening vigil for his predecessor Cardinal Francis George. He said,

> "We will hear in these days, as we have already, many well-deserved laudatory words about the Cardinal's life and ministry. His scholarship and razor-sharp incisive mind, his leadership in this country and abroad, his tenacity and courage in the face of great suffering and disability all merit our great admiration and respect. But, our Catholic tradition hesitates to let the past dominate these days of funeral liturgies. It considers such an approach short-sighted, so unequal to the totally other reality taking place. Our funerals are not celebrations of one's life, a

nostalgic return to past glories. Rather, they focus on the Risen Christ presently active in our midst, whose power at work in us is able to accomplish far more than we ask and far more that we can imagine."

Cardinal Cupich is right. In order for us not to get stuck in the past or fear the future, the funeral rite needs to be a lens through which all in attendance can better see the compassion of God and the hope in God's promises. If celebrated well, the funeral liturgy can begin to transform despair into hope, and grief into belief in something greater than the pain of this moment. All of this becomes even more powerful if the minister has had the opportunity to meet with the deceased during the later stages of illness, incorporating these insights into the process. Also, many parishioners have spoken to Barbara about the music they'd like at their funerals, and to me about the funeral itself. As long as this isn't driven by a deep need to control, it can become a gentle way for the terminally ill to begin to prepare their loved ones for their own indwelling.

MEETING WITH YOUR FUNERAL OFFICIATE

After his mother's funeral, a parishioner wrote me a note that echoed the sentiments many families have expressed through the years. His mother had battled many challenges in her life, dealing with them as best she could. Rather than glossing over these issues, I framed them in relation to the wounds life dealt her, connecting the dots that are often invisible to those too close to the situation. Instead of glorifying her into some fictionalized version of herself, I focused on the ways God had been working in her life through all of it, acknowledging her vulnerability and losses as part and parcel of the human experience we call life. I talked about a merciful God who loves us through our struggles, understands our pain, and is ready to embrace, to heal, to raise up.

Her son wrote me this note after the services:

"Thank you for helping us see my mother in new and healing ways. When I met with you, you parsed her life with compassion and understanding. You helped my brother and me see her with new eyes. I'm still not sure how you did it. Thank you for the amazing homily that put her life before us in a dignified but honest way. You helped us to understand her, to see the totality of her story that we were largely blind to before."

It is extremely important for families to meet in advance with the spiritual leader who will officiate at the funeral. I've found that many people suddenly begin to worry about heaven and hell, begin to see that the "heaven" of naïve faith, in which the deceased is "somewhere up there, smiling down at us," just doesn't satisfy. So, I map out the "Three Phases of Living" represented in the Journey of the Soul and walk families through it, not as a tidy roadmap to the afterlife, but as a sweeping expression of a mystery and a promise given to us by God.

After outlining the Three Phases of Living, we gently explore the life of the deceased. Family stories are usually complicated, often steeped in assumptions about one another's motivations, decisions, and actions. The family, raw with grief, sometimes harbors regrets, secret resentments, and disappointments. Many times these very human feelings are buried beneath the glorification of the deceased, causing guilt over the complex unacknowledged feelings or unresolved issues of the past. An insightful guide can compassionately validate the family story, anchoring it firmly in God, connecting the dots between woundedness and healing, vulnerability and courage, challenges and triumphs, and pointing out how God was actively present in all of it.

When you meet with your spiritual leader to plan the funeral service, be open about the family story, about the ups and downs of phase one of the deceased's journey. I encourage the family to embrace the entirety of it through the lens of mercy and compassion – as God does. I ask about childhood and adolescence, young adulthood and adulthood and, if the deceased lived a long life, about the elder years. I remind them that suffering empties us, but if we let God's love fill us, it's *his* strength that manifests as courage, *his* love expressed in each act of kindness, even if we don't realize it. Because if they can't recognize the hand of God in the life of the deceased, they also won't be able to understand where God is in their *own* lives. When we miss this important point we end up having to wait until our own deaths to finally see the ways in which God has always been there for us. This conversation is an opportunity to help families "see." It isn't any surprise that Jesus spent so much time healing the blind. Spiritual blindness is still a very real part of our human experience.

After they share their insights about the deceased, I talk with them about the mystery of Death and Resurrection - phases 2 and 3 of the Journey of the Soul. This helps families better imagine "where their loved one is now," and what this means in terms of their relationship and their faith.

If your spiritual guide is unable to guide you down this road to a deeper understanding, go back and revisit the earlier chapters in this book. Take an "EKG" of the deceased's life. Look at the high and low points, the early wounds and losses. How did the person move through it? On her/his own power? Where was God in it, working quietly behind the scenes? Extend a lens of gentleness, of mercy, of healing, and embrace the lovely human brokenness that makes us all who we are.

Let's look at each movement of the Funeral Rite. While we'll be exploring this through the Catholic Christian tradition, the basic progression is the same in the ritual observances of many faiths. Like the movements of a symphony, together they provide a cohesive, inter-related, and meaningful whole.

THE FIRST MOVEMENT: VIGIL TIME

The time between the moment of death and the funeral is what I call the Vigil Time, designed to commemorate and celebrate the First Phase of the Journey of the Soul (Birth, Living and Dying of the deceased). This "between time" serves an important purpose – helping family and friends begin to come to terms with the new reality before them, encouraging the acceptance of death as a natural part of life. Loved ones usually gather informally in the home, offering support to one another. Neighbors and friends bring food, flowers, or other gifts of sustenance or comfort.

A more formal part of this vigil time is known as the "wake," where the deceased is laid out and family and friends come to pay respects. I strongly encourage families, whenever possible, to have an open casket at the wake, as this brings greater closure to this rite of passage. As you stand before the deceased, there's a profound realization that the soul, the very essence of the person has left the body. It is also a sobering reminder of our own mortality.

The wake also serves as a healing vehicle for solace and story-telling. Photographs can be shared and displayed, favorite music played. It's a chance to celebrate the living and dying of the deceased: her/his high points, accomplishments, endearing qualities, as well as the challenges. The "calling hours" offer a unique opportunity to share recollections of the deceased from a variety of perspectives. These stories allow those in attendance to embrace the totality of the person who's died. It is a time of tears and of laughter. Words of endearment, love, forgiveness, and prayer can be expressed.

When I officiate at the Wake Service I encourage the family to begin to view the life story of the deceased in a larger context, to step back enough to consider the ways in which God cared for and supported him or her across a lifetime. I always ask, "What qualities did she/he possess? " and encourage people to respond aloud. It's heartening to hear people's impressions, some expected, some surprising. As guests share I facilitate and deepen the recollections, asking, "In what sense? " or "Tell us more about that." In telling the person's story, formally or informally, aspects of the person that the family didn't know are often revealed. This helps all in attendance put together a richer puzzle of the person's life than the one they knew. Often people provide examples that elicit nods, affirmations, and laughter. Others call forth tissues and bitter-sweet reflection. I always say, "Tears are the elevators of the emotions, moving them from the mind and rooting them deeply in the heart." Once rooted in the heart, powerful emotions can be surrendered to God, embraced, and healed. All of this becomes a healing balm for loved ones.

After people present the deceased's qualities, I raise questions such as, "Where did her courage come from? Her kindness? How was she able to overcome life's difficulties? How was she consoled and healed during disappointment and loss? How was she able to forgive life, self, and others? How did she love out of her suffering?" In other words, whether or not anyone recognized it, the deceased had a fertile patch inside through which God worked. This is the truth I strive to lead people toward. Scripture is read, to allow people to hear how God speaks to us in this moment. Prayers are recited. I also ask those in attendance to pray for the family, that their faith be deepened.

The Wake Service includes an Invitation to Prayer: *My brothers and sisters, we believe that all the ties of friendship and affection which knit us as one throughout our lives do not unravel with death...* What a message of hope – that the bonds of friendship and caring do not die with our loved ones. For me, this passage is the bridge leading us to the second ritual movement – the funeral service, priming the pump for a greater realization of the ways God is working not only in the journey of the deceased, but in our own lives as well.

THE SECOND MOVEMENT: THE FUNERAL SERVICE

The funeral service is designed to celebrate and commemorate the Second Phase of Living (Resurrection, Purification, and Oneness). Its main focus is on what God is doing, *right now*, for the deceased. Rather than glorifying the humanity of the loved one, which takes us back to the past, the funeral liturgy shifts the focus to the present, to the God-relationship, to the broader reality that we mostly fail to see. It is a celebration steeped in sacred paradox - our grieving hearts hold on to past memories, while our faith draws us toward a new reality. This creative tension points to the mystery at the heart of it – God's power and promise to raise the deceased (and all of us) from the dead. Do we believe it? The funeral liturgy, ripe with symbolism, links God's promises to our present reality.

THE GATHERING RITE – THE RECEPTION OF THE BODY

When we gather at the entrance of the Church, the presider of the service greets us, with these or similar words: *"The grace and peace of God our Father, who raised Jesus from the dead, be with you always."* The minister's presence reminds us that we are entering into a sacred time and space, inviting us to surrender the deceased to a merciful God.

The presider then **sprinkles** the coffin or urn with holy water to help us remember that the deceased was baptized and that he/she is God's son/daughter, having the privilege of calling God, "Abba - Father." This sprinkling echoes the words in the first letter of John 3: 1-2:

> *See the love the father has bestowed on us that we may be called the children of God. Yet so we are. The reason the world does not know us is that it did not know him. Beloved, we are God's children now; what we shall be has not yet been revealed. We do know that when it is revealed we shall be like him, for we shall see him as he is.*

As the presider sprinkles, he says: *"In the waters of baptism_____ died with Christ and rose with him to new life. May he/she now share with him eternal glory."*

The **baptismal pall** (a white sheet) is placed over the coffin or the urn by the family members, harkening back to the white garment worn at baptism. It reminds us that our beloved is being wrapped in God's love and mercy. The sprinkling and the placing of the pall are powerful symbols of what God has done and continues to do for the deceased. The coffin or urn is brought to the front of the church, led by the cross bearer and the minister, the casket accompanied by pall-bearers, and followed by family and other mourners. Most important events – graduations, weddings, the Olympics – begin with a procession. These dignified movements connote a "before and after" and bring a serious sense of anticipation for what is about to take place. The funeral procession is, in many ways, a display of opposites – made up of the living and the dead, the weak and the strong, the young and the old, the past and present - highlighting what I call "the escalator of life." It reminds us that the escalator moves pretty fast. And then, once the casket or urn is in place and everyone is seated, the service begins.

THE EULOGY

Over time I've come to believe that the eulogy is best placed right after the Opening Prayer. More commonly, the eulogy is presented after communion, but I've found this to be less effective. The movement of the mass takes us into mystery - the congregation is moved from the surface of life to deeper, larger truths. Inserting the eulogy late in the service abruptly brings us back to the Vigil time, reminiscing about phase one of the deceased's journey. Once that happens, it's difficult, if not impossible, to touch back into that mysterious deep inexpressible knowing brought about through the course of the liturgy. I prefer to have congregants leave the service changed, touched by this great mystery experienced in the mass – and to carry it with them into the world, uninterrupted. Also, when the eulogy is presented up front, it is the perfect closing of the Vigil time, before we drop into the liturgy.

The nature and content of the eulogy also needs to be considered. Barbara and I have served at over a thousand funerals together and have heard as many eulogies. Sadly, the eulogy is often a one-sided caricature of a person, glorifying their strong points and overlooking their struggles. Sometimes it takes on the tone of a humorous "roast," providing comic relief. This is unfortunate because it takes people out of the transformative nature of the service. And, think about it – is that the way we'd like to be remembered? By humorous quips and anecdotes? Is there anything of greater consequence to be considered here? The complex dichotomy of the deceased, a glimpse of the "both/and" that made them human. Their relationships. A sense of the role God played in his/her life across the years. These deeper questions not only touch into the essence of the deceased, but lead those in attendance to ask the same questions of themselves.

So, I tell families to select the eulogist carefully – someone who has the maturity and insight to see beneath the surface, and the courage and compassion to reflect on the deceased through the eyes of God. Most importantly, the eulogist should be able to recognize and point out how God was working throughout the life of the deceased.

LITURGY OF THE WORD

The Bible is sometimes seen as an ancient text written for an ancient audience. But, consider what St. Paul said in Hebrews 4:1:

> *The word of God is living and effective, sharper than any two edged sword, penetrating even between soul and spirit, joint and marrow, and able to discern reflections and thoughts of the heart."*

The readings, one from the Old Testament, a Psalm (which should be sung), a New Testament reading, and especially the Gospel, speak directly to us in real time, revealing profound truths about life and death that speak to this particular moment. As you listen to the sacred word, the question is, "What is God saying about the life, death, and resurrection of the deceased? And what does the Word proclaimed reveal about our own Journeys of the Soul? If you choose a family member or friend to read, be sure that they're well-prepared, emotionally composed, and that they understand the huge responsibility of being God's mouthpiece.

HOMILY

In order for the minister to touch the hearts of those in attendance, to speak with authority to the particular circumstance of this death, it's important to spend time with the family and friends before the service. Certainly the minister can speak, in a general way, about what God is doing for the deceased, and, in fact, for all of us. But, at this time when emotions are raw, the bereaved long to hear about what God is doing in the journey of the deceased and in their lives, now.

For me, the objective of the homily is to provide those in attendance with a "God lens" through which they see their beloved deceased in a new light. The familiar takes on another dimension, as they connect the person they have known, with the person God sees. This can only be done well when the minister and family share openly.

Recently a woman wrote me a thank you note after her brother's funeral service. She wrote:

Dear Father Lynch,

I am writing to say thank you for your delicate and caring handling of my brother's funeral service. All who attended, family and friends alike, said they felt as if you were speaking directly to them. It was an eclectic group of practicing Catholics, lapsed Catholics, devout Protestants, and even a few agnostics, but you managed to touch the hearts of each and every person. Your words held a message that deeply affected all of us.

This is what we want the bereaved to take away. A transformative experience that helps them see the deceased - and death itself - through eyes of faith.

After hearing the homily, those in attendance should understand that the deceased has the opportunity to be embraced by a merciful God, raised up, healed and made whole – a process of becoming one with their God. And where is God? Within each one of us. (See Chapter 12: The Indwelling of God) Loved ones begin to realize that the deceased, now in full union with God, will therefore dwell *within them* as well. This invites all to open their hearts in a greater way to God, allowing the deceased to love them in new and deeper ways – the way none of us can in the flesh. I always tell families, "You don't have to wait until your own death to know that the person who has died now loves you in a greater way, and wants to lead you closer to the God that they're one with." Regardless of our past, or of the nature of the relationship, none of us have to be held prisoner by a past story.

PRAYER OF THE FAITHFUL

Here, prayers of intention or petition are offered. Your minister may provide you with prayers to choose from, or guidelines that will assist the family in personalizing these prayers. We always pray for the deceased, that he or she may open his/her heart to God's invitation: *Will you let me love you?* We also include prayers for everyone assembled, that their faith be deepened, for all those who have been wounded by life, that they be healed. Not only do we pray for the family of the deceased, but for anyone in attendance that has lost a loved one. A family member or members can offer these prayers, with the congregation responding to each petition: *Lord, hear our prayer.*

LITURGY OF THE EUCHARIST

The first part of the Liturgy of the Eucharist is the "preparation of the gifts." I always invite family members to bring forward the gifts of bread and wine, as a gesture of setting the table for those assembled, as well as for all of those who have gone before us in faith. Sharing a meal is the way we mark rites of passage and commemorate important occasions. It's perhaps the most common way of demonstrating love to those we care for. Just as they've gathered to share meals with their loved ones in the flesh, I want them to understand that dining at the Lord's table *is* the family table, in a universal and timeless sense.

The following phrases are used in our various Eucharistic Prayers when we remember the dead and commend them to our Father. This invitation to the Lord's table is extended to:

all who died in my friendship
all who have died in the peace of my Christ.
all who were united with my Son in a death like His
all who have fallen asleep in the hope of the resurrection
all who have gone before us with the sign of faith
all the dead whose faith I alone have known
all who have died in my mercy...

It's important to note that *everyone* has died in God's mercy. These inclusive phrases show how God's heart is bigger than we can even imagine. He wants to invite all of us to His heavenly banquet so that he can share his gift of love and life eternal. For this, we give thanks.

Once the table is set, we prepare with grateful hearts for the Eucharistic meal.

In fact, the word "Eucharist" means to give thanks to God for what He has, is, and will do for us every day of our lives. We especially give thanks to God, our Father for "breaking the bonds of death and manifesting the Resurrection."

Remember, the Eucharist is considered a "heavenly banquet" in which those who are assembled are united with those who have gone before us and have consented to open their hearts to the compassionate love of God. When we gather, we are in communion with the Lord Jesus, the Blessed Virgin Mary, the Apostles, Martyrs, the Saints, and our deceased loved ones whose hearts are becoming more one with God's heart. We call this the communion of saints. When our hearts are open in faith to receive the intimacy of God's love through his body and blood, we're also open to receive the love of all those who have gone before us in Christ.

FINAL COMMENDATION AND THE GIFT OF FAREWELL

The final commendation is a last goodbye, professed as loved ones entrust the deceased to God. It's an opportunity to express powerful emotions and make closure before the committal (burial). I find, that for loved ones, the final commendation emphasizes the approaching physical separation and the reality of the "new normal" before them. There are two prayers the priest may recite:

1.) *Before we go our separate ways, let us take leave of our brother/sister. May our farewell express our affection for him/her; may it ease our sadness and strengthen our hope. One day we shall joyfully greet him/her again when the love of Christ, which conquers all things, destroys even death itself.*

or...

2.) *Trusting in God, we have prayed together for _____ and now we come to the last farewell. There is sadness in parting, but we take comfort in the hope that one day we shall see _____ again and enjoy his/her friendship. Although this congregation will disperse in sorrow, the mercy of God will gather us together again in the joy of his kingdom. Therefore let us console one another in the faith of Jesus Christ.*

The coffin or urn is once again sprinkled with holy water as a reminder of our baptism – affirming that just as we became a new creation in the baptismal waters, we're now becoming a new creation in and through our death (phase 2).

The coffin is also incensed, reverencing the dignity of the body, and as a reminder that the body was a temple of the Holy Spirit. The assembly is also incensed because they too are temples of the Holy Spirit—God dwells within them.

During this time, just before the "Song of Farewell" I ask the family to call to mind the deceased. I tell them, "If you have something to say, say it. If there's something to forgive, forgive it, for none of us has it together. If he/she gave you a special gift, or made your journey a little easier, thank him/her for it. And, if you can, use words of endearment to say goodbye." I also remind them that they must say goodbye to what has been in order to welcome what is now being birthed in them – the living and loving presence of the deceased. The person who has passed and been raised up now shares the same desire as God: *Will you let me love you?*

I invite others in attendance who may not have made closure with someone they love who died, to do so now. Then the Song of Farewell is sung: *May the choirs of Angels come to greet you, may they lead you to paradise. And may they lead you to the holy city, the new and eternal Jerusalem.*

THE THIRD MOVEMENT: THE COMMITTAL SERVICE - THE BURIAL

The Committal Service is designed to celebrate and commemorate the Third Phase of Living (The Resurrection of the Body and Life Eternal.) It is a short service that is all about leave-taking. It is a reminder that the world we know will some day evolve into a "new heaven and a new earth," we will be birthed into a glorified body, and live in love with all, forever. This perhaps is the greatest mystery of all, one steeped in hope, and symbolized by the body being returned to the earth. It is a concrete reminder that phase 1 is over, that phase 2 is underway, and that phase 3 will be glorious, beyond our ability to even imagine it.

If these three movements – the wake, the funeral, and the committal - are done with careful preparation and great care the results can be life-changing. Those who remain turn from the grave with a new hope, rooted deeply in faith in the power of God's love yesterday, today, and tomorrow.

351

CHAPTER 32

Grief Work: Healing and New Life

OFTEN, WHEN BARBARA and I discuss the aftermath of death, I remind her that when someone you love dies, he or she is raised up, made whole, and given back to loved ones left behind. Her *"Yeah but"* response inspired by an old Motown Song is always the same. Looking at me, she'll sigh, shake her head and say, "Yeah but...there ain't nothing like the real thing..."

And she's right. We humans know what we know, and we want what we want. A voice, a smile, a touch, an embrace. Sharing the good things of life, side by side.

Author and theologian C.S. Lewis, after the death of his beloved wife Helen (whom he referred to as H), says the same thing in his powerful book, *A Grief Observed*: "I know that the thing I want is exactly the thing I can never get. The old life, the jokes, the drinks, the arguments, the lovemaking, the tiny, heartbreaking commonplace. On any view whatever, to say, 'H is dead,' is to say, "All that is gone."

The theological explanation of the indwelling of the deceased loved one, while certainly preferable to "dead is dead," does little to relieve the grief we feel. Even when we leave the grave with deeper faith – a faith matured through suffering – we'll still, inevitably, experience the gnawing ache of loss. All of the false hopes that arose throughout treatment, the unfulfilled dreams, future plans that will never be realized – all of these losses become an excruciatingly heavy burden to bear.

That burden, however, pales in comparison to losing the *embodiment* of a relationship we were deeply invested in – more than invested in – a relationship that had become part and parcel of who we are. A piece of us has died as well. What's left is a gaping rupture in our hearts. This is the first fact that the bereaved have to deal with.

THE PARADOX OF GRIEF

The debilitating sadness experienced by the grieving is wrought with not only conflicting emotions, but with seemingly incongruent realities. There's a sense of loss so great that it's hard to put one foot in front of the other. At the same time, after a long debilitating illness, there may be a feeling of relief. The person you loved is no longer suffering. But isn't there some self-interest mixed in with that? This death delivered a welcome end to the sleepless nights, the ceaseless responsibilities and physical demands of care-giving, the constant challenges of medical bills, appointments, tests, hospital stays. This realization generates both guilt and anxiety. When a loved one dies suddenly, in the mainstream of life, the deceased likely suffered less, but was robbed of the ability to say goodbye and make closure. The bereaved are thrust onto the Path of Suffering, forced to walk this alone.

Another dichotomy is the fact that your loved one is *dead* and, at the same time, alive in a whole new way. You embrace the belief that your beloved is one with God and therefore dwelling within you, but wonder how to reconcile that with the overwhelming sense of loss and loneliness you're experiencing. And then there's the "unfinished business" of your relationship with the deceased. No relationship is perfect. Each comes with unresolved conflicts and challenges. These kinds of loose ends lure us into the old "what if" and "if only" thinking that can hold us prisoners of our past stories. Or, instead, we rewrite the story, making our beloved into a saint, remembering only the good. Our perceptions and memories of the deceased become fictionalized. Sadly, this skewed view prevents us from surrendering our beloved to God in his or her totality.

Again, I point to C.S. Lewis, who expresses this so well: "For, as I have discovered, passionate grief does not link us with the dead but cuts us off from them. This became clearer and clearer. It is just at those moments when I feel least sorrow – getting into my morning bath is usually one of them – that H. rushes upon my mind in her full reality, her otherness. Not, as in my worst moments, all foreshortened and patheticized and solemnized by my miseries, but as she is in her own right."

Moving Forward

As you move through the grieving process, walk gently. Engage in regular spiritual practice. Practice letting go. Find a soul partner, if you can, to help you anchor this experience in God. One, two, ten times a day, ask God to heal this gaping wound, and for the faith to believe in God's healing. Pray for the grace to forgive life for ripping someone from your heart, or others who may have hurt you throughout this process. (Remember, holding on to any unforgiveness blocks God's healing power.) Pray for a sense of gratitude, even in the face of great loss. Mindfully give thanks for one small gift each day – the sun on your face. A child's laughter. A tender memory. Go inside yourself to access the indwelling of God, and with it, the love of the person who passed.

These 2 facts – that, on the one hand, the person you love is *dead*, and on the other hand, that this person you love is alive in the Lord – these must be integrated. In the beginning, the first fact will naturally dominate. Over time, in faith, you can begin to allow the second fact of your loved one's indwelling to prevail. Without this transition, it will be difficult to move forward in a life-giving way.

Remember, this is a process. You'll need to push yourself to put one foot in front of the other, and remember – on your own power you may not be able to accomplish it. But, if you place your pain, your loneliness, your seeming lack of purpose squarely in God's hands, you can count on *God's* strength, on *God's* power, on *God's* grace and merciful love to carry you through.

Fortunately, there are many, many excellent books and resources on grief. You might join a bereavement group – many churches have them, as do hospitals and community groups. Spend time with family and loved ones. Practice doing little things with great love. Volunteer. Give back. Reach out. Don' let our wounded ego-selves bully us. When we love out of our suffering, we will become the face of God to others.

And, as you are doing the work of grieving, your loved one is working as well. As St. Therese said in a letter to her friend Fr. Roulland, shortly before her death, "The Lord, in His infinite mercy, will have opened His kingdom to me and I shall be able to draw His treasures in order to grant them liberally to the souls dear to me. I really count on not remaining inactive in heaven. What attracts me to the homeland of heaven is the Lord's call, the hope of loving Him finally as I have so much desire to love Him, and the thought that I shall be able to make Him loved by a multitude of souls who will bless Him eternally." Therese knew that her work in heaven would be to lead her loved ones closer to the God she was one with. Your deceased loved ones will do the same for you. As Jesus said in John 12:24: *Amen, amen, I say to you, unless a grain of wheat falls to the ground and dies, it remains just a grain of wheat; but if it dies, it produces much fruit.* The "fruit" of your loved one's death is this: to lead you closer to the God you're already one with.

As you open yourself to this pulsation of God (and the deceased), little by little, a moment here, a moment there, you'll begin to feel alive again. Moments turn to minutes, and minutes to hours. Hours to days, to weeks, to months. To years. In time, a new creation will emerge. You'll be able to look back with a smile, with an understanding of the gifts received. Wiser. More compassionate. You'll become a "wounded healer" sharing the depth of your experience and all you've learned about life and love with others when they, or someone they love receive death's calling card. In time a new creation will emerge. For God promised us:

He will wipe every tear from their eyes, and there shall be no more death or mourning, wailing or pain, for the old order has passed away. – Revelation 21:4

Behold, I make all things new. – Revelation 21:5

Credits, Permissions, and Acknowledgments

Scripture passages have been taken from *Saint Joseph Edition of The New American Bible*. The Old Testament of the New American Bible copyright 1970 by the Confraternity of Christian Doctrine (CCD), Washington, D.C. (Books of 1 Samuel to 2 Maccabees copyright 1969); Revised New Testament of the New American Bible copyright 1986 CCD, Revised Psalms of the New American Bible copyright 1991 CCD, Catholic Book Publishing Corp., New York, N.Y. Used with permission.

Chapter 1

POPE FRANCIS, https://w2.vatican.va/content/francesco/en/audiences/2013/documents/papa-francesco_20131030_udienza-generale.html

MERTON, Thomas, "The Road Ahead" from THOUGHTS IN SOLITUDE, Copyright © 1958 by the Abbey of Our Lady of Gethsemani. Copyright renewed 1986 by the Trustees of the Thomas Merton Legacy Trust. Reprinted by permission of Farrar, Straus and Giroux.

Chapter 2

SAINT THERESE OF LISIEUX, *Story of a Soul*, trans. John Clarke, O.C.D. Copyright (c) 1975, 1976, 1996 by Washington Province of Discalced Carmelites ICS Publications 2131 Lincoln Road, N.E. Washington, DC 20002-1199 U.S.A. www.icspublications.org 265 p. Used with permission.

DECHANE, Robert, *Continuing Journey*, (Mustang, OK: Tate Publishing LLC, 2011) 38-39 p. Used with Permission.

Chapter 4

LANGAGER, Chad, *Sportingcharts.com*, 2015

DE MELLO, Anthony, Excerpt(s) from THE WAY TO LOVE: THE LAST MEDITATIONS OF ANTHONY DE MELLO by Anthony De Mello, copyright © 1991 by Gujarat Sahitya Prakash of Anand, India. Used by permission of Doubleday, an imprint of the Knopf Doubleday Publishing Group, a division of Penguin Random House LLC. All rights reserved.

Chapter 8
EINSTEIN, Albert, http://alberteinstein.info/vufind1/Record/EAR 000028196

DE MELLO, Anthony, Excerpt(s) from THE WAY TO LOVE: THE LAST MEDITATIONS OF ANTHONY DE MELLO by Anthony De Mello, copyright © 1991 by Gujarat Sahitya Prakash of Anand, India. Used by permission of Doubleday, an imprint of the Knopf Doubleday Publishing Group, a division of Penguin Random House LLC. All rights reserved.

POPE FRANCIS: *Homily,* September 4, 2003

POPE FRANCIS: *Homily,* Casa Santa Marta, November 18, 2014

Chapter 10
Three quotes from pp.45, 72, 72-73 from THE DARK NIGHT OF THE SOUL by GERALD G. MAY, M.D. COPYRIGHT © 2004 BY GERALD G. MAY. Reprinted by permission of HarperCollins Publishers.

CAMPBELL, Joseph, *The Hero with a Thousand Faces,* (Princeton, NJ: Princeton University Press, 1972) 25 p. Used with Permission of the Joseph Campbell Foundation.

Chapter 11
KUZEL, Cathy, *The Ruby Slippers Principle* (http://cathykuzel.com/the-ruby-slippers-principle/)

MAY, Gerald G. M.D., *The Dark Night of the Soul,* (New York, NY: HarperCollins Publishers, Inc., 2004) 45 p. Used with Permission

KEATING, Thomas, https://www.youtube.com/watch? v=p-Q9ql0Pqo0

FACTCHECKING INJUSTICE FACTS https://factcheckinginjustice-facts.wordpress.com/2012/01/16/asmaa-al-hameli/

RUMI, *It's Rigged,* From *Love Poems from God: Twelve Sacred Voices From the East and West* by Daniel Ladinsky, (New York, NY: Penguin Group, 2002) Used with Permission.

Chapter 12
Man's Search for Meaning, by Victor E. Frankl, Copyright © 1959, 1962, 1984, 1992 by Victor E. Frankl
Reprinted by permission of Beacon Press, Boston 37 p.

I am a Rock
Words and Music by Paul Simon
Copyright © 1965 Paul Simon (BMI)
International Copyright Secured All Rights Reserved
Used by Permission
Reprinted by Permission of Hal Leonard LLC

ALEXANDER, Eben, M.D. *Proof of Heaven,* (New York, NY: Simon & Schuster, ©2012) 71 p. Reprinted with permission of Simon & Schuster, Inc.

SAINT THERESE OF LISIEUX, *Story of a Soul,* trans. John Clarke, O.C.D. Copyright (c) 1975, 1976, 1996 by
Washington Province of Discalced Carmelites ICS Publications 2131 Lincoln Road, N.E.
Washington, DC 20002-1199 U.S.A. www.icspublications.org Used with permission.

Chapter 13

LANGFORD, Joseph, *Mother Teresa's Secret Fire* (Huntington, IN: Our Sunday Visitor Publishing Division, 2008) 282-283 p. Used with permission.

From YOUR GOD IS TOO SMALL by J.B. Philips Copyright ©1952 by J.B. Philips; copyright renewed 1998 by Vera May Phillips. Reprinted with the permission of Touchstone, a division of Simon & Schuster, Inc. All Rights Reserved

SAINT JOHN PAUL II, *Dives in Misercordia (DM,7)* http://w2.vatican.va/content/john-paul-ii/en/encyclicals/documents/hf_jp-ii_enc_30111980_dives-in-misericordia.html, November 30, 1980

KASPER, Cardinal Walter, *Mercy: The Essence of the Gospel and the Key to Christian Life*, (Mahwah, NJ: Paulist Press, 2014) 139 p.

POPE FRANCIS, *The Joy of the Gospel: Apostolic Exhortation, Evangelii Gaudium*, 2013

POPE FRANCIS, *Apostolic Letter: Misericordia et misera*, https://w2.vatican.va/content/francesco/en/apost_letters/documents/papa-francesco-lettera-ap_20161120_misericordia-et-misera.html November 20, 2016

Chapter 14

CHAPIN, E.H., *Discourses on the Beatitudes* (Edwin Hubbell), 1814-1880. p. 36.

NOUWEN, Henri J.M., *The Wounded Healer,* (New York, NY: Image Books, Penguin/Random House, 1979) 45 p. Used with permission.

ROHR, Richard, *Things Hidden: Scripture as Spirituality, p. 25* used with permission from Franciscan Media

POPE FRANCIS, http://vaticanfiles.org/en/2013/09/65-the-pope-francis-dogma-god-is-present-in-every-persons-life/

KIERKEGAARD, Soren, *Upbuilding Discourses in Various Spirits,* translated by H.V. Hong & E.H. Hong (Princeton University Press, 1993)

Chapter 15
CASEY, Michael, *Fully Human, Fully Divine* © 2004 Liguori Publications liguori.org 181 p. Used with permission. All rights reserved.

MAY, Gerald G. M.D., *The Dark Night of the Soul,* (New York, NY: HarperCollins Publishers, Inc., 2004) 72-73 p. Used with Permission

POPE FRANCIS, http://www.catholicnews.com/services/englishnews/2016/doubts-about-faith-should-spur-deeper-study-prayer-pope-says.cfm November 23, 2016

Chapter 16
SIMMONS, Philip, *Learning to Fall: The Blessings of an Imperfect Life,* (New York, Toronto, London, Sydney, Auckland: Bantam Books, 2002) 8 p. Used with permission, Kathryn Field

NOUWEN, Henri J.M., Excerpt(s) from REACHING OUT: THE THREE MOVEMENTS OF THE SPIRITUAL LIFE by Henri Nouwen, copyright © 1975 by Henri J. M. Nouwen. Copyright renewed © 2003 by Sue Mosteller, Executor of the Estate of Henri J.M. Nouwen. Used by permission of Doubleday, an imprint of the Knopf Doubleday Publishing Group, a division of Penguin Random House LLC. All rights reserved.

Chapter 17

RAHNER, Karl, S.J., *The Need and the Blessing of Prayer*, Copyright 1997 by Order of Saint Benedict. Liturgical Press, Collegeville, Minnesota: 39, 45, 46, 47 p. Used with permission.

Excerpt from *Mother Teresa's Secret Fire* ©Fr. Joseph Langford, (Huntington, IN: Our Sunday Visitor Publishing Division, 2008) 191-192 p. www.osv.com, Used by Permission

POPE BENEDICT, *cf. Dei Verbum 25*, https://w2.vatican.va/content/benedict-xvi/en/speeches/2005/september/documents/hf_ben-xvi_spe_20050916_40-dei-verbum.html September 16, 2005

Chapter 18

POPE FRANCIS, https://twitter.com/pontifex/status/495494769213063171?lang=en

UNITED CONFERENCE OF CATHOLIC BISHOPS, *The Roman Missal*, (New Jersey; Catholic Book Publishing Corp, 2011) 644 p.

UNITED CONFERENCE OF CATHOLIC BISHOPS, *The Roman Missal*, (New Jersey; Catholic Book Publishing Corp, 2011) 644-645 p.

Chapter 20

Saint Theresa of Calcutta, *Nobel Lecture* www.nobelprize.org Dec. 11, 1979

Saint Theresa of Calcutta, Do small things with great love, *Catholic News Service, Conference of Catholic Bishops* Sept. 4, 2016 www.catholicnews.com

Chapter 21

ILIBAGIZA, Immaculee, *Left to Tell* (Carlsbad, CA, Hay House, Inc, 2006), 93 p. 196-197 p.

LEWIS, C.S., *Essay from BBC Radio Broadcast*, http://www.pbs.org/wgbh/questionofgod/ownwords/mere2.html

GANDHI, Mahatma, http://www.bbc.co.uk/worldservice/learningenglish/movingwords/shortlist/gandhi.shtml

KING, Martin Luther, Jr. *(Loving your Enemies – Sermon – Christmas, 1957, Dexter Avenue Baptist Church)* Reprinted by arrangement with The Heirs to the Estate of Martin Luther King Jr., c/o Writers House as agent for the proprietor New York NY © 1957 Dr. Martin Luther King, Jr. © renewed 1985 Coretta Scott King

Chapter 23
Daughters of St. Paul, Charles de Foucauld's "Prayer of Abandonment" from *Journey of the Spirit* p.78 by Cathy Wright, Copyright ©2015, Cathy Wright, Daughters of St. Paul. Used with Permission

POPE JOHN XXIII, *Overlook Much, Correct a Little*, edited by Hans-Peter Rothlin (Hyde Park, New York, NY, New City Press 2007) 51 p. Used with permission

THE GRACE IN DYING: HOW WE ARE TRANSFORMED SPIRITU-ALLY AS WE DIE by KATHLEEN DOWLING SINGH. Copyright ©1998 by Kathleen Dowling Singh. Courtesy of HarperCollins Publishers.

Chapter 26
TWYCROSS, Robert, http://www.life.org.nz/euthanasia/euthanasiafaq1

IHRIG, Tim, http://www.theatlantic.com/health/archive/2015/02/death-in-america-is-getting-more-painful/385230/

SAINT FRANCIS DE SALES, *Be at Peace* http://www.integratedcatholi-clife.org/2012/03/daily-catholic-quote-from-st-francis-de-sales/

Chapter 28

UNITED STATES CONFERENCE OF CATHOLIC BISHOPS, *Ethical and Religious Directives for Catholic Health Care Services, Fifth Edition*, 2009, Part Five, Items 56, 58, 26p., 27p. Used with permission

BENSON, Richard, C.M., Ph.D., S.T.D., *Embracing Our Dying: A Project of the California Catholic Conference*, Articles IV, V, VI
Used with permission

POPE JOHN PAUL II, *Life Sustaining Treatment and the Vegetative State*, March 20, 2004

Chapter 30

NATIONAL CONFERENCE OF CATHOLIC BISHOPS, *The Roman Missal*, (New Jersey, Catholic Book Publishing Corp. 2011), 492 p. Used with permission

The Pastoral Care of the Sick: the Rites of Anointing and Viaticum, 194.p Used with permission

Chapter 31

RUTHERFORD, Richard with BARR, Tony, *The Death of a Christian: The Order of Christian Funerals*, (Collegeville, Minnesota, The Liturgical Press, 1980) 3 p. Used with permission

CUPICH, BLASE Cardinal, zenit.org/articles/archbishop-cupich-s-homily-at-wake-for-cardinal-george/April 22, 2015

NATIONAL CONFERENCE OF CATHOLIC BISHOPS, *Order of Christian Funerals*, (New Jersey, Catholic Book Publishing Corp. 1998) 27 p. Used with permission

NATIONAL CONFERENCE OF CATHOLIC BISHOPS, *Order of Christian Funerals*, (New Jersey, Catholic Book Publishing Corp. 1998) 81p
Used with permission

NATIONAL CONFERENCE OF CATHOLIC BISHOPS, *The Roman Missal*, (New Jersey, Catholic Book Publishing Corp. 2011) 621p, 513p, 507p, 501p, 513p. Used with permission

NATIONAL CONFERENCE OF CATHOLIC BISHOPS, *Order of Christian Funerals*, (New Jersey, Catholic Book Publishing Corp. 1998) 89p.
Used with permission

Chapter 32
LEWIS, C.S. *A Grief Observed*, (New York, N.Y., Harper Collins, 1996) 25 p., 54-55 p. © copyright CS Lewis Pte Ltd 1961 Used with Permission

CLARKE, JOHN, O.C.D. *General Correspondence Volume Two* Copyright (c) 1988 by Washington Province of Discalced Carmelites, ICS Publications, Used with Permission

TREECE, PATRICIA, *Mornings with Saint Therese: 120 Daily Readings* (Manchester, New Hampshire, Sophia Institute Press, © 1997, 2015) 160-161 p. Used with Permission